Transboundary Diseases of Cattle and Bison

Editors

ELIZABETH J. PARKER
CHARLES P. FOSSLER
CARLA L. HUSTON

VETERINARY CLINICS OF NORTH AMERICA: FOOD ANIMAL PRACTICE

www.vetfood.theclinics.com

Consulting Editor
ROBERT A. SMITH

July 2024 • Volume 40 • Number 2

ELSEVIER

1600 John F. Kennedy Boulevard • Suite 1800 • Philadelphia, Pennsylvania, 19103-2899

http://www.vetfood.theclinics.com

**VETERINARY CLINICS OF NORTH AMERICA: FOOD ANIMAL PRACTICE Volume 40, Number 2
July 2024 ISSN 0749-0720, ISBN-13: 978-0-443-29386-3**

Editor: Taylor Hayes
Developmental Editor: Varun Gopal

Veterinary Clinics of North America: Food Animal Practice (ISSN 0749-0720) is published in March, July, and November by Elsevier Inc., 360 Park Avenue South, New York, NY 10010-1710. Subscription prices are $281.00 per year (domestic individuals), $100.00 per year (domestic students/residents), $298.00 per year (Canadian individuals), $356.00 per year (international individuals) $100.00 per year (Canadian students), and $165.00 (international students). For institutional access pricing please contact Customer Service via the contact information below. To receive student/resident rate, orders must be accompanied by name of affiliated institution, date of term, and the signature of program/residency coordinator on institution letterhead. *Clinics* subscription prices. All prices are subject to change without notice. **POSTMASTER:** Send address changes to *Veterinary Clinics of North America: Food Animal Practice*, Elsevier Health Sciences Division, Subscription Customer Service, 3251 Riverport Lane, Maryland Heights, MO 63043. Customer Service (orders, claims, online, change of address): Elsevier Health Sciences Division, Subscription **Customer Service, 3251 Riverport Lane, Maryland Heights, MO 63043. Tel: 1-800-654-2452 (U.S. and Canada); 314-447-8871 (ouside U.S. and Canada). Fax: 314-447-8029. E-mail: journalscustomerservice-usa@elsevier.com (for print support); journalsonlinesupport-usa@elsevier.com (for online support).**

Reprints. For copies of 100 or more, of articles in this publication, please contact the Commercial Reprints Department, Elsevier Inc., 360 Park Avenue South, New York, NY 10010-1710. Tel.: 212-633-3874; Fax: 212-633-3820; E-mail: reprints@elsevier.com.

Veterinary Clinics of North America: Food Animal Practice is covered in *Current Contents/Agriculture, Biology and Environmental Sciences, MEDLINE/PubMed (Index Medicus),* and *Excerpta Medica.*

Contributors

CONSULTING EDITOR

ROBERT A. SMITH, DVM, MS
Diplomate, American Board of Veterinary Practitioners; Veterinary Research and Consulting Services, LLC, Greeley, Colorado; Veterinary Research and Consulting Services, LLC, Stillwater, Oklahoma, USA

EDITORS

ELIZABETH J. PARKER, DVM
Consultant, Parker AgriInsight Solutions, LLC, College Station, Texas, USA

CHARLES P. FOSSLER, DVM, PhD
Beef Specialist, Veterinary Epidemiologist, National Animal Health Monitoring System, USDA:APHIS:VS:CEAH, Fort Collins, Colorado, USA

CARLA L. HUSTON, DVM, PhD
Diplomate, American College of Veterinary Preventive Medicine (Epidemiology); Professor and Beef Extension Veterinarian, Director of Enhanced Clinical Education Program, College of Veterinary Medicine, Mississippi State University, Mississippi State, Mississippi, USA

AUTHORS

WILLIAM AMANFU, DVM, MSc
International Veterinary Consultant, Accra, Ghana

MUHAMMAD JAVED ARSHED, DVM, MSc, PhD
Global Project Coordinator, Food and Agriculture Organization of the United Nations, Rome, Italy

JONATHAN ARZT, DVM, MPVM, PhD
Diplomate, American College of Veterinary Pathologists; Veterinary Medical Officer, Foreign Animal Disease Research Unit, Agricultural Research Service, U.S. Department of Agriculture, Plum Island Animal Disease Center, Greenport, New York, USA

PAOLO CALISTRI, DVM
Veterinary Officer, Veterinary Operations Center for Epidemiology, Programming, Information (COVEPI), Istituto Zooprofilattico dell'Abruzzo e del Molise "G. Caporale" or Experimental Zooprophylactic Institute of Abruzzo and Molise "G. Caporale", Teramo, Italy

CRISTINA W. CUNHA, DVM, MS, PhD
Veterinary Medical Officer, United States Department of Agriculture, Agricultural Research Service, Animal Disease Research Unit, Pullman, Washington State, USA

FRANCESCA DALL'ACQUA, BSc (Zoology), MSc (Veterinary Epidemiology)
Researcher, Veterinary Operations Center for Epidemiology, Programming, Information (COVEPI), Istituto Zooprofilattico dell'Abruzzo e del Molise "G. Caporale" or Experimental Zooprophylactic Institute of Abruzzo and Molise "G. Caporale", Teramo, Italy

ALESSANDRA DI GIUSEPPE, DVM
Researcher, Veterinary Operations Center for Epidemiology, Programming, Information (COVEPI), Istituto Zooprofilattico dell'Abruzzo e del Molise "G. Caporale" or Experimental Zooprophylactic Institute of Abruzzo and Molise "G. Caporale", Teramo, Italy

DARIA DI SABATINO, DVM
Veterinary Officer, Veterinary Operations Center for Epidemiology, Programming, Information (COVEPI), Istituto Zooprofilattico dell'Abruzzo e del Molise "G. Caporale" or Experimental Zooprophylactic Institute of Abruzzo and Molise "G. Caporale", Teramo, Italy

BARBARA DROLET, MS, PhD
Research Entomologist, Agricultural Research Service, United States Department of Agriculture, Manhattan, Kansas, USA

AHMED EL IDRISSI HAMZI, DVM, PhD
International Animal Health Expert, Rome, Italy

THOMAS HAIRGROVE, BS, DVM, PhD
Professor and Extension Veterinary Specialist, Department of Animal Science, Texas A&M AgriLife Extension, College Station, Texas, USA

CARLA L. HUSTON, DVM, PhD
Diplomate, American College of Veterinary Preventive Medicine (Epidemiology); Professor and Beef Extension Veterinarian, Director of Enhanced Clinical Education Program, College of Veterinary Medicine, Mississippi State University, Mississippi State, Mississippi, USA

AKIKO KAMATA, DVM, MSc
Animal Health Officer, The Food and Agriculture Organization of the United Nations, Rome, Italy

J. BRIAN KIMBLE, PhD
Molecular Biologist, Foreign Arthropod-Borne Animal Diseases Research Unit, National Bio and Agro-Defense Facility, USDA, ARS, Manhattan, Kansas, USA

JUAN LUBROTH, BA, MSc, DVM, PhD, ACVPM, AVES (Hons)
Former Chief Veterinary Officer, Food and Agriculture Organization of the United Nations, Doctor of Veterinary Medicine, Lubroth One Health Consultancies, Casaprota, Italy

NICK LYONS, MA, VetMB, MSc, PhD, MRCVS
Diplomate of the European College of Bovine Health Management; Veterinary Head of TB Policy Advice, Animal Health and Welfare Advice, Service Delivery Directorate, Animal and Plant Health Agency (APHA), Strathearn House, Perth, United Kingdom

MARIANA MARRANA, DVM
Programme Manager, Preparedness and Resilience Department, World Organisation for Animal Health, Paris, France

BETHANY MCGREGOR, MS, PhD
Research Entomologist, Agricultural Research Service, United States Department of Agriculture, Manhattan, Kansas, USA

DANA MITZEL, PhD
Molecular Biologist, Foreign Arthropod-Borne Animal Diseases Research Unit, National Bio and Agro-Defense Facility, USDA, ARS, Manhattan, Kansas, USA

LEELA NORONHA, DVM, PhD
Researcher, Foreign Arthropod-Borne Animal Diseases Research Unit, National Bio and Agro-Defense Facility, USDA, ARS, Manhattan, Kansas, USA

ANGELA M. PELZEL-MCCLUSKEY, DVM, MS
Equine Epidemiologist, United States Department of Agriculture, Animal and Plant Health Inspection Service, Veterinary Services, Fort Collins, Colorado, USA

JUERGEN A. RICHT, DVM, PhD
Professor, Diganostic Medicine, Pathobiology, Kansas State University, Manhattan, Kansas, USA; Department of Veterinary Tropical Diseases, Faculty of Veterinary Science, University of Pretoria, Onderstepoort, South Africa

MO SALMAN, DVM, MPVM, PhD
Diplomate, American College of Veterinary Preventive Medicine (DIP ACVPM); Professor of Preventive Veterinary Medicine and Infectious Animal Diseases, Animal Population Health Institute of College of Veterinary Medicine and Biomedical Sciences, Colorado State University, Fort Collins, Colorado, USA; Food and Agriculture Organization of the United Nations, Rome, Italy

MICHAEL W. SANDERSON, DVM, MS
Diplomate, American College of Veterinary Preventive Medicine (Epidemiology); Department of Diagnostic Medicine/Pathobiology, Kansas State University, Director, Center for Outcomes Research and Epidemiology, Manhattan, Kansas, USA

KYLE SHIPMAN, DVM
Animal Programs Division Director, Indiana State Board of Animal Health, Indianapolis, Indiana, USA

CAROLINA STENFELDT, DVM, PhD
Scientist, Foreign Animal Disease Research Unit, Agricultural Research Service, U.S. Department of Agriculture, Plum Island Animal Disease Center, Greenport, New York, USA; Department of Diagnostic Medicine/Pathobiology, Kansas State University, Manhattan, Kansas, USA

PETE D. TEEL, BS, MS, PhD
Regents Professor, Department of Entomology, Texas A&M AgriLife Research, College Station, Texas, USA

JESSIE D. TRUJILLO, DVM, PhD
Senior Research Associate, Diganostic Medicine/Pathobiology, Kansas State University, Manhattan, Kansas, USA

SHERRILYN H. WAINWRIGHT, DVM, MPH
Veterinary Epidemiologist, United States Department of Agriculture, Animal and Plant Health Inspection Service, Veterinary Services, Fort Collins, Colorado, USA

BRETT WEBB, DVM, PhD
Diplomate, American College of Veterinary Pathologists; Veterinary Pathologist, North Dakota State University, Veterinary Diagnostic Laboratory, Fargo, North Dakota, USA

JOHN B. WELCH, PhD
Entomologist, New World Screwworm Expert, Action Programs, International Services, Animal and Plant Health Inspection Service, United States Department of Agriculture, College Station, Texas, USA

JOHN WENZEL, DVM
Veterinarian, Extension Animal Sciences and Natural Resources, New Mexico State University, Las Cruces, New Mexico, USA; Southwest Veterinary Services, Silver City, New Mexico, USA

KELLI KIRTLEY WERLING, DVM
Senior Director of Operations, Animal Programs Division, Indiana State Board of Animal Health, Indianapolis, Indiana, USA

WILLIAM C. WILSON, PhD
Research Microbiologist, Foreign Arthropod-Borne Animal Diseases Research Unit, National Bio and Agro-Defense Facility, USDA, ARS, Manhattan, Kansas, USA

VALENTINA ZENOBIO, DVM
Researcher, Veterinary Operations Center for Epidemiology, Programming, Information (COVEPI), Istituto Zooprofilattico dell'Abruzzo e del Molise "G. Caporale" or Experimental Zooprophylactic Institute of Abruzzo and Molise "G. Caporale", Teramo, Italy

Contents

Foot-and-mouth disease (FMD) is a viral infection of livestock that is an important determinant of global trade in animal products. The disease causes a highly contagious vesicular syndrome of cloven-hoofed animals. Successful control of FMD is dependent upon early detection and recognition of the clinical signs, followed by appropriate notification and response of responsible government entities. Awareness of the clinical signs of FMD amongst producers and veterinary practitioners is therefore the key in protecting US agriculture from the catastrophic impacts of an FMD outbreak. This review summarizes key clinical and epidemiologic features of FMD from a US perspective.

Transboundary animal disease (TAD) investigations are conducted routinely across the United States to rule out diseases of significant economic, trade, and/or food security importance. Established protocols exist for TAD investigations and disease response based on national and international policy; however, now more than ever, private practitioners may be called upon to assist in these investigations and response activities and may play an important role in communications, sample collection, and disease surveillance. Successful implementation of disease investigation and response, with or without vaccination, requires a collaborative effort between regulatory officials, industry groups, private practitioners, and producers.

The threat of foreign animal diseases is steadily increasing. Veterinary practitioners play a vital role in a community's preparedness for, response to, and recovery from a foreign animal disease outbreak. This article examines the steps a practitioner needs to take to become ready to have a role in disaster readiness and response. Resources exist to provide the practitioner with tools needed to transition their normal daily activities to a larger integrated response. The knowledge and skills used by practitioners in disaster management lead to a more effective and efficient response to a foreign animal disease.

> Transboundary animal diseases are defined by the Food and Agriculture Organization (FAO) of the United Nation's Emergency Prevention System as those diseases that are of significant economic, trade and/or food security importance, which can easily spread to other countries and reach epidemic proportions, and where control/management including exclusion requires cooperation among several countries. The Global Framework for the Progressive Control of Transboundary Animal Diseases represents a platform of the FAO and World Organisation for Animal Health to engage regional sub-regional organizations and national veterinary authorities in developing and monitoring progress in animal disease management efforts.

> Vesicular stomatitis (VS) is a vector-borne livestock disease caused by either VS New Jersey virus or VS Indiana virus. The disease circulates endemically in northern South America, Central America, and Mexico and only occasionally causes outbreaks in the United States. During the past 20 years, VS outbreaks in the southwestern and Rocky Mountain regions occurred periodically with incursion years followed by virus overwintering and subsequent expansion outbreak years. Regulatory response by animal health officials prevents spread from lesioned animals and manages trade impacts. Recent US outbreaks highlight potential climate change impacts on insect vectors or other transmission-related variables.

> Lumpy skin disease (LSD) is a contagious non-zoonotic viral disease of cattle. The disease raises great concern due to the recent rapid spread toward free countries and reoccurrence in countries where control and preventive measures had achieved eradication. Deep nodules involving skin, subcutaneous tissue, and occasionally muscles are localized mostly in the head, neck, perineum, genitalia, udder, and limbs. LSD can cause large economic losses mainly because of the decline in milk production and the decrease in hide value, in addition to the ban of movement of animals and animal products.

> Contagious bovine pleuropneumonia (CBPP) is one of the six high impact diseases for which currently World Organisation for Animal Health (WOAH) has established an official procedure for recognition of disease-free status for trade purposes. Although its exact distribution, incidence, and impact

have not been well established, the disease is known to be endemic in sub-Saharan Africa, where it has a severe socio-economic impact on people's livelihoods. Control or elimination of the disease can be achieved by various strategies including vaccination, movement control, and stamping-out. Due to many factors, countries in sub-Saharan Africa are still struggling with this disease, compromising continental and global eradication. In this review, basic epidemiologic features and clinical signs of CBPP are presented and disease control challenges, particularly in endemic countries, are briefly discussed.

Rift Valley fever (RVF) is a zoonotic viral disease that affects domestic and wild ruminants such as cattle, sheep, goats, camels, and buffaloes. Rift valley fever virus (RVFV), the causative agent of RVF, can also infect humans. RVFV is an arthropod-borne virus (arbovirus) that is primarily spread through the bites of infected mosquitoes or exposure to infected blood. RVFV was first isolated and characterized in the Rift Valley of Kenya in 1931 and is endemic throughout sub-Saharan Africa, including Comoros and Madagascar, the Arabian Peninsula (Saudi Arabia and Yemen), and Mayotte.

Transboundary incursions of ticks and tick-borne pathogens are ever present concerns for US cattle industries. Global trade in livestock and wildlife, historic and emerging transboundary issues with endemic tick populations and pathogens, and migratory bird flyways are pathways of concern. Transboundary challenges are presented for the Asian longhorned tick and *Theileria orientalis* Ikeda, for 2 cattle fever tick species [*Rhipicephalus (Boophilus) annulatus* and *R (B) microplus*] and *Babesia bigemina* and *B bovis*, and for the tropical bont tick and *Ehrlichia ruminantium*.

Reemerging and notifiable diseases of cattle and bison continue to pose potential risks to their health and lives and affecting production and the livelihoods of producers. It is essential to understand the clinical presentation of these diseases to watch for possible incursions and infections and to immediately report your suspicions to your State and Federal Animal Health Officials. Three of these reemerging and notifiable diseases of cattle and bison, malignant catarrhal fever, bluetongue virus, and New World screwworm, are presented in this article for increased awareness to consider as a differential if examinations present suggestive clinical signs.

Rinderpest is a highly contagious viral disease that affects ungulates such as cattle, buffalo, yak, and various wildlife species, leading to significant morbidity and mortality. The global eradication of rinderpest was successfully accomplished in 2011 through extensive vaccination efforts. Today, safeguarding against the re-emergence of rinderpest in animal populations is paramount. The Food and Agriculture Organization of the United Nations and the World Organisation for Animal Health are entrusted through a series of resolutions with the responsibility to prevent the re-emergence of rinderpest in animals.

VETERINARY CLINICS OF NORTH AMERICA: FOOD ANIMAL PRACTICE

Preface

Transboundary Diseases of Cattle and Bison

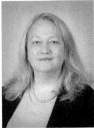

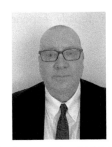

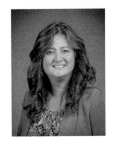

Elizabeth J. Parker, DVM   Charles P. Fossler, DVM, PhD   Carla L. Huston, DVM, PhD
Editors

Many veterinarians in the United States view animal diseases that are not present in the country, such as foot-and-mouth disease, as foreign animal diseases (FADs). In the international community, the preferred term is transboundary animal diseases (TADs). A disease that is foreign to one country may be endemic in another, so FADs is not a term applicable across the globe. The only disease that could be considered "foreign" to all countries is rinderpest, which was eradicated in 2011. TADs have significant trade, economic, or food security implications, can spread easily between countries, and can require cooperation among countries for control of the disease. This issue of *Veterinary Clinics of North America: Food Animal Practice* covers transboundary diseases of cattle and bison that can have a tremendous negative impact on producers and the veterinarians who serve them. Detrimental impacts can extend nationally, causing severe economic impacts, and for TADs that are zoonotic, significant public health consequences. The threat of TADs to North America has increased in recent years due to a more globalized society with frequent movement of livestock and livestock products between countries, and a concerning rapidly evolving distribution of relevant vectors. Reemerging and reportable diseases have become a more frequent concern in the United States and globally. A veterinarian's ability to diagnose endemic diseases and recognize TADs is a significant responsibility. Veterinarians can play a variety of roles during an outbreak, depending on the situation, and can substantially contribute to decreasing negative impacts to their clients, their practices, their communities, and our nation, by being able to assist with prevention, preparedness, surveillance, and response efforts.

Veterinarians are leaders in the communities they serve and contribute daily to national security and national/global food security. We are fortunate in the United States to have strong networks of producers, veterinarians, and state and federal

Vet Clin Food Anim 40 (2024) xiii–xiv
https://doi.org/10.1016/j.cvfa.2024.01.012
0749-0720/24/© 2024 Published by Elsevier Inc.

animal health officials. Training and infrastructure investments, geography, and effective responses in the past decades have enabled the US livestock herd to have very few to no-incursions of most of the diseases discussed in this issue. Rapid detection and ensuring you and your clients become prepared during periods when current disease conditions are stable will make a difference when an outbreak occurs.

We encourage veterinarians to familiarize themselves with the increasing TADs threats, work with your clients to prepare enhanced biosecurity plans, plan for your own business continuity, and work with your community, state, and national leaders to prepare for, prevent, and effectively, rapidly respond to TADs such as those discussed in this issue.

DISCLOSURES

The guest editors have no financial conflicts of interest and have nothing to disclose.

Elizabeth J. Parker, DVM
Parker AgriInsight Solutions LLC
College Station, TX 77840, USA

Charles P. Fossler, DVM, PhD
National Animal Health Monitoring System
USDA:APHIS:VS:CEAH
2150 Centre Avenue, Building B-2E7
Fort Collins, CO 80526, USA

Carla L. Huston, DVM, PhD
College of Veterinary Medicine
Mississippi State University
PO Box 6100
Mississippi State, MS 39762, USA

E-mail addresses:
eparker@parkeragriinsightsolutions.com (E.J. Parker)
charles.p.fossler@usda.gov (C.P. Fossler)
huston@cvm.msstate.edu (C.L. Huston)

Foot-and-Mouth Disease

Jonathan Arzt, DVM, MPVM, PhD[a], Michael W. Sanderson, DVM, MS[b],
Carolina Stenfeldt, DVM, PhD[a,c],*

KEYWORDS

- Foot-and-mouth disease • Foot-and-mouth disease virus • FMD • FMDV • Cattle
- Virus • Transboundary animal disease

KEY POINTS

- Foot-and-mouth disease (FMD) is a notifiable vesicular disease that spreads rapidly amongst cloven-hoofed animals. The lesions may be clinically indistinguishable from vesicular lesions of other etiologies.
- In the event of observing vesicular disease in any ungulate species in the United States, a practitioner or producer should immediately contact and notify the State Animal Health Official (SAHO) and U.S. Department of Agriculture Veterinary Services Area Veterinarian in Charge.
- The response to an FMD incursion in North America would involve culling of animals on infected premises and strict animal movement controls and quarantine measures; vaccination of susceptible animals would only be performed under specific scenarios.
- Successful control of an FMD outbreak is dependent upon early detection and appropriate notifications. Awareness of the clinical signs of FMD amongst producers and practitioners is critical for initiation of efficient control measures.

BACKGROUND

Foot and mouth disease (FMD) is a viral disease of cloven-hoofed animals that is caused by foot-and-mouth disease virus (FMDV; genus: *Aphthovirus,* family: Picornaviridae). It is a high-consequence transboundary animal disease and an outbreak in North America could have catastrophic impacts on the agricultural industry. FMD has not occurred in North America since an outbreak in Saskatchewan, Canada, in 1952,[1] preceded by northern Mexico in 1946,[2] and California, United States, in

[a] Foreign Animal Disease Research Unit, Agricultural Research Service, U.S. Department of Agriculture, Plum Island Animal Disease Center, PO Box 848, Greenport, NY 11944, USA; [b] Department of Diagnostic Medicine/Pathobiology, Kansas State University, Center for Outcomes Research and Epidemiology, 1800 Denison Avenue, Manhattan, KS 66502, USA; [c] Department of Diagnostic Medicine/Pathobiology, Kansas State University, 1800 Denison Avenue, Manhattan, KS 66502, USA
* Corresponding author. Foreign Animal Disease Research Unit, Agricultural Research Service, U.S. Department of Agriculture, Plum Island Animal Disease Center, PO Box 848, Greenport, NY 11944.
E-mail address: Carolina.Stenfeldt@usda.gov

Vet Clin Food Anim 40 (2024) 191–203
https://doi.org/10.1016/j.cvfa.2024.01.001
0749-0720/24/© 2024 Elsevier Inc. All rights reserved.

1929.[3] Currently, FMD is endemic in most of Asia and Africa. South America is FMD-free with or without vaccination, excepting Colombia and Venezuela where sporadic outbreaks have occurred within the past decade.[4]

There are 7 known serotypes of FMDV: O, A, C, Asia-1, and Southern African Territories (SAT)-1, -2, and -3.[5] FMDV serotypes were originally defined based on lack of serologic cross-reactivity; thus, infection by one serotype will not protect against subsequent infection by another. The antigenicity of the FMDV capsid is largely determined by the VP1 protein, which is 1 of 4 structural proteins encoded by the approximately 8 kb positive-sense RNA genome. Given the increased availability of genomic sequencing tools, FMDV VP1 sequencing has become the most common approach to characterizing FMDV strains for molecular epidemiology and outbreak investigations. However, recent works have demonstrated that full-genome length sequencing provides additional critical information pertaining to the origins and evolution of specific FMDV lineages, including historic and recent recombination events between heterologous viruses.[6–8] These genomic data provide important clues in the emergence and movement of new strains of FMDV which is useful in understanding and targeting control efforts. Genomic data are also necessary for assessing vaccine candidates against circulating or introduced strains.

CLINICAL PRESENTATION AND PATHOGENESIS

The classic clinical presentation of FMD in cattle consists of fever, lameness, and hypersalivation associated with painful vesicles in the oral cavity and areas of non-haired skin, including coronary bands, inter-digital clefts, and teats. The severity of the clinical signs can vary greatly depending on both host genetics and on viral strain properties. In general, domestic cattle bred for intensive production purposes in countries that are free of FMD are more susceptible to the clinical effects of FMD than indigenous breeds originating in FMD endemic regions. There is limited knowledge concerning FMDV infection of North American bison. One published study describes experimentally infected bison having high susceptibility and clinical lesions similar to those observed in cattle.[9] However, despite similar lesion distribution, the more stoic behavior of the bison resulted in less overt clinical signs such as lameness compared to the cattle that were included in the same investigation.[9]

Mortality due to FMD is low in adult animals, whereas juvenile animals may sporadically succumb to sudden death due to viral-associated myocarditis.[10] Such fatal cases may occur without vesicular lesions or other signs suggestive of FMD; thus, thorough clinical examination of adult animals in the herd is critical for correct diagnosis. FMDV transmits rapidly via direct contact (secretions and aerosols) between infected and susceptible animals and can also be transmitted passively through contaminated fomites. It has been reported that aerosolized FMDV can spread over considerable distances under certain climatic and atmospheric conditions.[11,12]

Foot-and-Mouth Disease Virus Pathogenesis

In cattle, the initial site of infection involves specific epithelial segments within the nasopharyngeal mucosa.[13–15] In contrast to pigs, cattle are highly susceptible to FMDV infection through inhalation, consistent with the primary infection site in the upper respiratory tract. In naïve animals, FMDV disseminates systemically through a phase of cell-free viremia, followed by secondary viral amplification at peripheral lesion sites.[16] The viremic phase is followed by a strong antibody-mediated immune response, with antibodies against structural FMDV proteins detectable in serum as early as 5 to 7 days after infection.[17] The characteristic vesicular lesions appear within approximately 2 to 5 days of virus exposure,[14,18] and are first observed as areas of blanched skin that develop into fluid-filled vesicles (**Fig. 1**). Vesicles often rupture within 24 hours and leave epithelial erosions or ulcers. FMD lesions typically heal within 5 to 10 days of appearance, but secondary bacterial infections at lesion sites

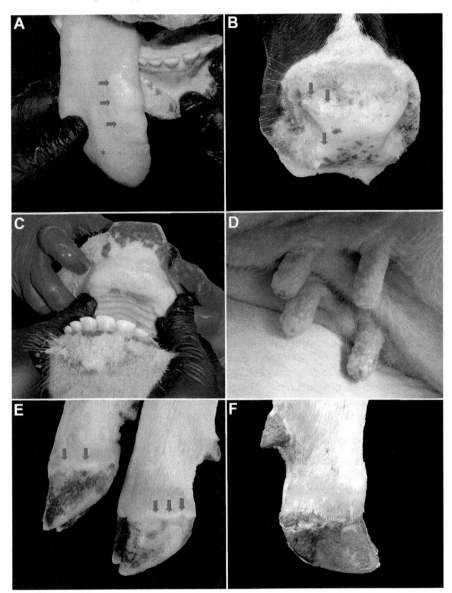

Fig. 1. Foot-and-mouth disease lesions in experimentally infected Holstein heifers. (*A*) Intact coalescent vesicles of the tongue (*arrows*) as well as an area of blanched tongue epithelium on the rostral tongue (*asterisk*), 4 days post infection (dpi). (*B*) Ruptured vesicles on muzzle (*arrows*) and hypersalivation, 4 dpi. (*C*) Erosion (sloughed vesicle) on the dental pad/hard palate, 4 dpi. (*D*) Multiple vesicles on the teats. 4 dpi. (*E*) Early-stage coronary band vesicles characterized by blanching and mild swelling (*arrows*), 4 dpi. (*F*) Late-stage coronary band lesion with sloughed epithelium, incomplete healing, and separation of the hoof wall, 17 dpi.

are common. Additionally, chronic sequela such as hoof deformities may arise as a consequence of coronary band lesions that cause separation of the hoof wall (see **Fig. 1**).

Foot-and-Mouth Disease Virus Persistence

Approximately 50% of cattle remain persistently infected with FMDV after the clinical phase, a condition commonly referred to as the FMDV carrier state, which may last for several months to years,[19,20] (Bertram M, Yadav S, Stenfeldt C, Delgado A, Arzt J. Extinction Dynamics of the Foot-and-Mouth Disease Virus Carrier State Under Natural Conditions. Frontiers in Veterinary Science. 2020). The 1 published investigation of FMDV infection in North American bison did not demonstrate FMDV persistence in that species.[9] However, that phase of the investigation comprised only 3 animals. The epidemiologic relevance of FMDV carriers remains controversial as there has been no demonstration of virus transmission from carriers under controlled experimental conditions.[19] Regardless, the FMDV carrier state is hugely important to control measures, as the prolonged existence of infected animals delays a nation's return to FMD-free status and may thereby favor depopulation or vaccination to slaughter over vaccination to live. Whereas a vaccination to live strategy would intend to leave vaccinated animals in the population, a vaccination to slaughter approach would intend for vaccinated animals to enter slaughter channels as scheduled for feedlots or earlier than otherwise scheduled for cow-calf and dairy herds to facilitate quicker removal of such animals from the population.[21]

Persistent FMDV infection can only be diagnosed by scraping of the upper respiratory tract mucosa using a specialized sputum cup, known as a "probang cup."[22] True shedding of virus in oronasal secretions is limited during FMDV persistence,[18,23] which likely explains the comparatively low level of contagion associated with FMDV carriers, and further explains why conventional swab samples are inadequate for diagnosis. The serologic response to infection is similar in FMDV carriers as in animals that successfully clear infection.[17,24] Detection or quantitation of antibodies against FMDV can therefore not be used to diagnose FMDV persistence. The FMDV carrier state can occur regardless of pre-occurring clinical FMD; thus, animals that are protected from FMD by vaccination may become subclinically infected and progress to become FMDV carriers without any visible signs of infection.

Detection of Foot-and-Mouth Disease Virus Infection

Definitive diagnosis of FMD cannot be made based on the clinical presentation alone. The most important differential diagnosis in bovines in North America is vesicular stomatitis (VS), which causes lesions that are indistinguishable from FMD. The key points for differentiation are (1) VS in cattle typically causes 1 or 2 vesicles, not generalized lesions, (2) VS occurs as sporadic individual cases (arthropod-borne transmission), whereas FMDV has high morbidity, with classical contagious disease transmission patterns, (3) VS may affect horses, which are not susceptible to FMD. Sloughed FMD vesicles may appear similar to lesions of other viral infections that cause oral erosions; thus, additional differentials include bovine herpes virus, bovine parapox virus, bovine viral diarrhea virus, malignant catarrhal fever, and possibly bluetongue virus. Physical trauma such as thermal or caustic burns can also cause lesions that resemble FMD. Overall, the host range, systemic generalization, and rapid transmission of FMD separate it from the listed differentials. Thus, vesicular or erosive lesions at multiple sites, in multiple animals, that do not include any equids should give a strong suspicion of FMD.

For clinical cases, the optimal diagnostic sample consists of vesicular epithelium or fluid. These samples contain massive quantities of virus that can be detected through real-time reverse transcriptase-polymerase chain reaction (RT-PCR) or antigen enzyme-linked immunosorbent assay (ELISA).[25] Clinically affected animals shed large amounts of virus in oronasal secretions through the first 7 to 10 days of infection. As the viremic phase is of shorter duration, detection of FMDV RNA in serum is less useful for diagnostic purposes. Detection of antibodies against FMDV structural or non-structural proteins in serum by ELISA can be utilized from approximately 14 days after infection. While antibodies against structural capsid protein can provide information regarding the serotype of the infecting virus, the non-structural proteins are conserved across serotypes. Animals that are vaccinated against FMD will have detectable antibodies against structural proteins, whereas detection of antibodies against non-structural proteins is suggestive of previous infection. That approach can therefore be used to detect evidence of prior infection in vaccinated animals, which may be an indicator of potential FMDV persistence.[25] However, this differentiating infected from vaccinated animals approach is imperfect and is dependent upon high-quality, purified vaccines.

FOOT-AND-MOUTH DISEASE VIRUS EPIDEMIOLOGY

The conventional wisdom that FMD is the most contagious disease on the planet is less than completely substantiated by scientific data. That said, the epidemiologic hallmarks of high morbidity and rapid spread within, and between, premises are important features of this disease in non-endemic settings.

Specifically, the basic reproduction number for within-herd transmission (R_0), which indicates the relative transmissibility of an agent defined as the estimated number of secondary cases caused by each primary case, is very high. Based on observations from experimental studies, it has been estimated at 176 (95% CI 80–388).[26] Model estimates based on data from the United Kingdom 2001 FMD epidemic provided a within herd R_0 estimate of 21 (95% CI 16–25).[27] These R_0 values suggest rapid spread through an infected herd. Some field data from endemic countries suggest that not all animals in an infected herd will become infected and that segregation and barriers may decrease within-herd transmission.[28] However, the background of pre-existing immunity from previous vaccination and/or infection significantly affects transmission and clinical signs in endemic settings. Model data based on UK data and US production systems suggest that in an FMD-free context, most or all animals on a farm will become infected.[29,30] Experimental data suggest that vaccination may substantially decrease the R_0 value within herds.[31]

Estimates for between-herd transmission of FMD are more modest, with R_0 likely in the range of 2 to 3 prior to implementation of control activities.[32] Transmission risk from local sources include direct contacts along fence lines, indirect contacts from people, vehicles, other fomites, wildlife, and aerosols. These sources are not easily distinguished in field data. Infected pigs are considered a greater risk for generating infectious aerosols; however, large feedlots may pose a similar risk.[33] This implies that proximity to pig holdings or large feedlots may increase the risk of airborne introduction of FMDV to neighboring farms. Additionally, the presence of pigs on farms with multiple animal species constitutes a risk as infected pigs generate greater quantities of infectious aerosols than both cattle and small ruminants.[34]

An increased risk of infection as distance to an infected premise (IP) decreases is consistently supported in published studies,[35–37] suggesting the importance of local transmission. The route of local transmission is generally not known but may involve movement of wildlife such as rodents, birds, scavengers, domestic pets, people, or aerosols. Increasing herd size may increase the risk for disease introduction, perhaps due to increased import rates and likely also increases the time period that the herd will be infectious.[29,38] Local herd density is also a risk for infection.[36,39–41]

Direct contacts resulting from movement of livestock between operations is a key method of transmission between farms and necessitates movement control (quarantine) during outbreaks to limit spread. Movement of latent and subclinically infected cattle can transfer infection between farms before any clinical signs are detectable. The structure of the US cattle industry results in movements of cattle over long distances, potentially resulting in new IPs far remote from the source of infection. Currently there are no quantitative estimates of the risk of movements, conditional upon the risk profile of the individual herd.

FOOT-AND-MOUTH DISEASE CONTROL AND ERADICATION
Herd Detection and Management

Early detection of FMD following a potential introduction to the United States is critical to mitigating impact. The magnitude of the 2001 outbreak in the United Kingdom is widely attributed to delayed detection.[42] Model data based on US scenarios suggest delayed detection increases the expected number of IPs and the duration of outbreaks.[43,44] Producers and practicing veterinarians are the front line for detection of the initial case of FMD. As such, awareness and training to recognize signs of FMD are critical.

In the event of observing or suspecting vesicular disease in any ungulate species, a practitioner or producer should immediately contact and notify the State Animal Health Official (SAHO) or the U.S. Department of Agriculture (USDA) VS Area Veterinarian in Charge (AVIC). These officials will determine the likelihood of FMD and the need for implementation of control measures. If a foreign animal disease such as FMD is suspected, a state-employed or USDA-employed Foreign Animal Disease Diagnostician (FADD) will be deployed to the premise for collection and submission of appropriate samples.[45] Samples for FMDV testing are sent to the Foreign Animal Disease Diagnostic Laboratory (NVSL-FADDL) at the Plum Island Animal Disease Center, NY. During an outbreak, NVSL-FADDL will continue to confirm detections of FMD on any premises not currently in a Control Area. To increase test capacity, subsequent samples may be sent to other USDA-approved laboratories that are part of the National Animal Health Laboratory Network.[46] Plans for control of FMD once introduced into the United States are described in the USDA Foot-and-Mouth Disease Response Plan.[46] The plan provides details of planned and potential control efforts by State and Federal officials. In the event of an outbreak, rapid tracing of contacts of infected farms is also important for control, particularly for decreasing the risk of large outbreaks.[44] The control plan in the United States would include some combination of movement controls, quarantine of infected farms, establishment of control areas around infected farms for focused control and surveillance efforts, and depopulation (stamping-out) of animals on infected farms. In some scenarios, a vaccination program may be instituted.

Enhanced biosecurity is an effective measure to prevent FMD incursion at the level of the individual herd. Practitioners should aid their clients in developing and implementing a routine biosecurity plan as part of daily herd management, as well as enhanced biosecurity and business continuity plans for the specific operation to be implemented in the event of a disease outbreak.[45] An optimal plan includes continuity of business including empirical recommendations regarding enhanced biosecurity to decrease risk of disease entry. Resources for implementation of enhanced biosecurity recommendations are available,[47] including appointing a biosecurity officer in charge, establishing a written plan, risk management, establishing a line of separation around the farm, as well as cleaning and disinfection. Recommendations also include disease monitoring or active observational surveillance (AOS) for FMD clinical signs in the herd. While AOS will be typically done by the producer to assist in detection of clinical animals as soon as possible, training by the veterinary practitioner will be critical for effective implementation. Logs of animals, people, and vehicle movements onto the farm are also collected to assist in early identification of risks.[45] An FMD outbreak in the United States will disrupt agriculture operations substantially. Implementation of Secure Beef Supply guidelines[47] are meant to control disease transmission risk, while allowing continuity of business for cattle operations.

Environmental Contamination and Disinfection

FMDV is a non-enveloped virus and is therefore resistant to alcohol-based disinfectants. However, the viral capsid is highly sensitive to both acidic and basic pH; thus any disinfectant with a pH below 6 or above 8 will effectively inactivate the virus.[48] A list of disinfectants approved for use against FMDV in farm settings is available from USDA- Animal and Plant Health Inspection Service.[49] Research from recent years has shown that FMDV RNA can be detected in environmental samples obtained in proximity of IPs, which could potentially complicate disinfection, but may enhance surveillance efforts.[50,51] Data on environmental survival of FMDV are sparse, but optimal environmental survival of FMDV is at near neutral pH, temperatures less than 20°C, and greater than 55% humidity, with longer survival on organic material compared to inanimate surfaces. Survival may commonly exceed 50 days in organic material with low temperature and high humidity while survival on inorganic surfaces is substantially shorter.[52] Experimental studies have shown that FMDV may remain infectious in carcasses stored at 4°C for as long as 11 weeks[53] while hot and dry climatic conditions would be expected to lead to rapid inactivation of the virus.[54]

Foot-and-Mouth Disease Vaccines

FMD vaccination is restricted in countries with official status as free of FMD.[55] A decision to deploy vaccination as part of FMD control measures in a country previously free of FMD may delay the timeline of regaining official status as free of FMD.[55,56] However, efficient use of vaccination may prevent critical losses as the number of animals culled may be reduced and outbreak duration may be decreased. Disease control, animal welfare, and economic impacts should be considered in evaluation of a decision whether to vaccinate during an outbreak in a previously free country.[57]

For control of FMD in endemic countries, conventional FMD vaccines based on adjuvanted inactivated virus are used in prophylactic vaccine programs or in response to outbreaks. The vaccine antigen needs to be closely matched to circulating viral strains for optimal protection,[25] which necessitates thorough knowledge of the epidemiologic situation for effective application. Conventional FMD vaccines are limited both in duration and breadth of induced immunity. Furthermore, vaccination does not prevent subclinical infection of the upper respiratory tract, and thereby potential persistent infection of exposed cattle. Despite these limitations, vaccination was an integral part of efficient FMD eradication in Europe[58] and has been critical for FMD control in South America[59] as well as in successful response efforts to more recent FMD incursions in Japan[60] and South Korea.[61] High-quality FMD vaccines are purified to remove any non-structural FMDV proteins from the formulation. This facilitates differentiation of vaccinated and previously infected animals by detection of antibodies against non-structural proteins in serum. Any vaccination implementation would require official identification of vaccinated animals to facilitate either subsequent depopulation/slaughter of vaccinates or post outbreak surveillance in a "vaccinate to live" scenario in order to regain official free status.

Ongoing efforts in research and development of FMD vaccines include utilization of modern vaccine platforms, such as virus-like particles, recombinant viruses, and vectored vaccines that may improve the protection offered by vaccination as well as reduce the inherent risks associated with large-scale manufacture of inactivated vaccines.[62] Presently, no such alternatives are commercially available for use.

DISCUSSION

FMD is an important transboundary animal disease that has not been detected in North America since 1952 and not in the US since 1929. However, maintaining preparedness and awareness of FMD is critical due to the highly contagious nature of the disease in naïve animal populations, and the implications on animal movements and international trade associated with a potential incursion. Practitioners and producers have important roles in early detection and control. Most importantly, recognition of febrile vesicular syndromes in livestock species should trigger appropriate sampling and notifications.[46]

In the event of an FMD outbreak in North America, initial control efforts would include quarantine and depopulation of infected herds, tracing of contacts, and movement controls. Depending largely on the extent of the outbreak, control efforts may involve vaccination of susceptible animals on surrounding premises, in addition to culling of animals on IPs. However, implementation of vaccination to control FMD is a complex decision, with potentially large benefits, but also potential for an extended time required to regain status as free of FMD. This decision would be made by government officials and would involve considering potential financial benefits as well as losses associated with disease control and loss of export markets.[56,57,63] The US Foreign Animal Disease Preparedness and Response Plan (FAD PReP) Strategy recommends focus on stamping out for small outbreaks, with transition to a vaccination program for larger regional outbreaks.[64] In the event of a large-scale outbreak involving multiple premises, resources available for depopulation and carcass disposal would likely be overwhelmed,[65–67] and such scenarios would thereby require a modified control strategy.[68] In cases where depopulation of infected premises cannot be carried out effectively, practitioners will need to support their clients in addressing resulting biosecurity and animal welfare concerns.

Subclinical phases of FMDV infection complicate diagnosis and control efforts. These syndromes include the pre-clinical phase of infection, also referred to as neoteric subclinical infection, during which animals shed virus and may transmit infection prior to the development of clinical signs. Infectious virus may remain in the upper respiratory tract of convalescent animals for durations of months to years through what is commonly referred to as the FMDV carrier state.[19,20,69] Additionally, vaccinated animals that are exposed to the virus may progress from neoteric subclinical infection to persistent infection in the absence of any clinical signs of disease.[14,18] The epidemiologic relevance of FMD carriers is somewhat controversial. Although it is clear from experimental investigations that any potential contagion associated with such animals is indeed low, the high numbers of carriers that are present in a population following an outbreak may compensate for a low probability of transmission at the individual animal level. More importantly, as FMDV carriers constitute a distinct category of infected animals, the presence of such animals in the national herd would affect trade status, and would not be tolerated if pursuing an FMD-free status.

FMD continues to be one of the most important determinants of global trade of animal products, as FMD-endemic nations are restricted from trade with FMD-free regions. North America has remained FMD-free for over 7 decades, predominantly through biosecurity practices and border controls. Consequences of any FMD outbreak in North America would be substantial; however, the scale of impact could be mitigated from billions to millions of USD, through rapid detection and response by livestock producers and veterinarians.

CLINICS CARE POINTS

- The classic clinical presentation of FMD in cattle and bison is a syndrome of vesiculo-erosive lesions in the oral cavity and areas of non-haired skin (feet, muzzle, teats), fever, hypersalivation, lameness.
- The observation of vesicular lesions or erosions in oral cavities or on the feet of multiple animals in a herd should always trigger diagnostic testing to exclude FMD and immediate notification to the State Animal Health Officials and USDA AVIC.
- FMD is clinically indistinguishable from other vesicular diseases such as Vesicular Stomatitis, and diagnosis by detection of FMDV genome in vesicular epithelium or oronasal secretions is required to confirm diagnosis.
- If an FMD incursion is suspected, sample collection and submission for diagnostic testing will be performed by a Foreign Animal Disease Diagnostician
- Successful management of an FMD outbreak requires effective control measures that can only be initiated by appropriate government veterinary officials.
- Private practitioners and producers have a critical role in early detection of cases; early recognition of FMD by clinical and epidemiologic attributes is the most important measure to mitigate the scope and impact of an outbreak.
- Practitioners should support their clients in creating enhanced biosecurity plans as well as active observational surveillance and business continuity plans, which will be critical for continued operation in the event of an FMD outbreak.
- Effective control of an FMD outbreak in FMD-free regions requires a complex, multifaceted approach including depopulation, quarantine, movement control, enhanced biosecurity, and disinfection; the precise combination of response measures will be determined by responding government authorities and will depend on the extent and specific nature of the ongoing outbreak.
- In the event of an outbreak, practitioner involvement in effective implementation of biosecurity and disease monitoring will minimize dissemination and facilitate control of disease introduction risk through early detection of FMD on individual farms. These approaches will maximize business continuity.

DISCLOSURE

The authors have no financial interests to disclose.

ACKNOWLEDGMENT

This work was supported by U.S. Department of Agriculture, Agricultural Research Service (USDA-ARS) Current Research Information System Project 1940- 32000-064-00D (Arzt), as well as USDA-ARS grant 58-8064-9-019 (Sanderson) and USDA-APHIS grants AP22VSSP0000C020 and AP21VSSP0000C035 (Sanderson).

REFERENCES

1. Sellers RF, Daggupaty SM. The epidemic of foot-and-mouth disease in Saskatchewan, Canada, 1951-1952. Can J Vet Res 1990;54(4):457–64.
2. Dusenberry W. Foot and Mouth Disease in Mexico, 1946-1951. Agric Hist 1955; 29(2):82–90.
3. Mohler JR and Snyder R. The 1929 outbreak of foot-and-mouth disease in southern California, 1930, US Department of Agriculture. Available at: https://books.google.com/books/about/The_1929_Outbreak_of_Foot_and_mouth_Dise.html?id=mqgoAAAAYAAJ.
4. Rivera AM, Sanchez-Vazquez MJ, Pituco EM, et al. Advances in the eradication of foot-and-mouth disease in South America: 2011-2020. Front Vet Sci 2022;9: 1024071.
5. Knowles NJ, Samuel AR. Molecular epidemiology of foot-and-mouth disease virus. Virus Res 2003;91(1):65–80.
6. Brito B, Pauszek SJ, Hartwig EJ, et al. A traditional evolutionary history of foot-and-mouth disease viruses in Southeast Asia challenged by analyses of nonstructural protein coding sequences. Sci Rep 2018;8(1):6472.
7. Bachanek-Bankowska K, Di Nardo A, Wadsworth J, et al. Reconstructing the evolutionary history of pandemic foot-and-mouth disease viruses: the impact of recombination within the emerging O/ME-SA/Ind-2001 lineage. Sci Rep 2018; 8(1):14693.
8. Fish I, Stenfeldt C, Spinard E, et al. Foot-and-Mouth Disease Virus Interserotypic Recombination in Superinfected Carrier Cattle. Pathogens 2022;(6):11.
9. Rhyan J, Deng M, Wang H, et al. Foot-and-mouth disease in North American bison (Bison bison) and elk (Cervus elaphus nelsoni): susceptibility, intra- and interspecies transmission, clinical signs, and lesions. J Wildl Dis 2008;44(2): 269–79.
10. Arzt J, Baxt B, Grubman MJ, et al. The pathogenesis of foot-and-mouth disease II: viral pathways in swine, small ruminants, and wildlife; myotropism, chronic syndromes, and molecular virus-host interactions. Transbound Emerg Dis 2011; 58(4):305–26.
11. Gloster J, Blackall RM, Sellers RF, et al. Forecasting the airborne spread of foot-and-mouth disease. Vet Rec 1981;108(17):370–4.
12. Brown E, Nelson N, Gubbins S, et al. Airborne Transmission of Foot-and-Mouth Disease Virus: A Review of Past and Present Perspectives. Viruses 2022;14(5).
13. Arzt J, Pacheco JM, Rodriguez LL. The early pathogenesis of foot-and-mouth disease in cattle after aerosol inoculation: identification of the nasopharynx as the primary site of infection. Vet Pathol 2010;47(6):1048–63.
14. Stenfeldt C, Hartwig EJ, Smoliga GR, et al. Contact Challenge of Cattle with Foot-and-Mouth Disease Virus Validates the Role of the Nasopharyngeal Epithelium as the Site of Primary and Persistent Infection. mSphere 2018;(6):3.
15. Stenfeldt C, Eschbaumer M, Pacheco JM, et al. Pathogenesis of primary foot-and-mouth disease virus infection in the nasopharynx of vaccinated and non-vaccinated cattle. PLoS One 2015;10(11):e0143666.
16. Arzt J, Juleff N, Zhang Z, et al. The pathogenesis of foot-and-mouth disease I: viral pathways in cattle. Transbound Emerg Dis 2011;58(4):291–304.
17. Stenfeldt C, Heegaard PM, Stockmarr A, et al. Analysis of the acute phase responses of Serum Amyloid A, Haptoglobin and Type 1 Interferon in cattle experimentally infected with foot-and-mouth disease virus serotype O. Vet Res 2011; 42(1):66.

18. Stenfeldt C, Eschbaumer M, Rekant SI, et al. The foot-and-mouth disease carrier state divergence in cattle. J Virol 2016;90(14):6344–64.

19. Stenfeldt C, Arzt J. The Carrier Conundrum; A Review of Recent Advances and Persistent Gaps Regarding the Carrier State of Foot-and-Mouth Disease Virus. Pathogens 2020;9(3).

20. Hayer SS, Ranjan R, Biswal JK, et al. Quantitative characteristics of the foot-and-mouth disease carrier state under natural conditions in India. Transbound Emerg Dis 2018;65(1):253–60.

21. Foot-and-Mouth disease vaccination policy in the United States, October 2020 (2020).

22. Sutmoller P, Gaggero A. Foot-and mouth diseases carriers. Vet Rec 1965;77(33): 968–9.

23. Stenfeldt C, Lohse L, Belsham GJ. The comparative utility of oral swabs and probang samples for detection of foot-and-mouth disease virus infection in cattle and pigs. Vet Microbiol 2013;162(2–4):330–7.

24. Eschbaumer M, Stenfeldt C, Rekant SI, et al. Systemic immune response and virus persistence after foot-and-mouth disease virus infection of naive cattle and cattle vaccinated with a homologous adenovirus-vectored vaccine. BMC Vet Res 2016;12:205.

25. WOAH. Manual of Diagnistic Tests and Vaccines for Terrestrial Animals 2019. 381 Foot-and-Mouth Disease. 2022. p. 433-464.

26. Orsel K, Bouma A, Dekker A, et al. Foot and mouth disease virus transmission during the incubation period of the disease in piglets, lambs, calves, and dairy cows. Prev Vet Med 2009;88(2):158–63.

27. Chis Ster I, Dodd PJ, Ferguson NM. Within-farm transmission dynamics of foot and mouth disease as revealed by the 2001 epidemic in Great Britain. Epidemics 2012;4(3):158–69.

28. Hutber AM, Kitching RP. The role of management segregations in controlling intra-herd foot-and-mouth disease. Trop Anim Health Prod 2000;32(5):285–94.

29. Cabezas AH, Sanderson MW, Volkova VV. Modeling Intervention Scenarios During Potential Foot-and-Mouth Disease Outbreaks Within U.S. Beef Feedlots. Front Vet Sci 2021;8:559785.

30. Mielke SR, Lendzele S, Delgado AH, et al. Patterns of foot-and-mouth disease virus detection in environmental samples in an endemic setting. Front Vet Sci 2023; 10:1157538.

31. Orsel K, de Jong MC, Bouma A, et al. The effect of vaccination on foot and mouth disease virus transmission among dairy cows. Vaccine 2007;25(2):327–35.

32. Perez AM, Ward MP, Carpenter TE. Control of a foot-and-mouth disease epidemic in Argentina. Prev Vet Med 2004;65(3–4):217–26.

33. Coffman MS, Sanderson MW, Dodd CC, et al. Estimation of foot-and-mouth disease windborne transmission risk from USA beef feedlots. Prev Vet Med 2021; 195:105453.

34. Donaldson AI, Alexandersen S, Sorensen JH, et al. Relative risks of the uncontrollable (airborne) spread of FMD by different species. Vet Rec 2001;148(19):602–4.

35. McLaws M, Ribble C, Martin W, et al. Factors associated with the clinical diagnosis of foot and mouth disease during the 2001 epidemic in the UK. Prev Vet Med 2006;77(1–2):65–81.

36. Bessell PR, Shaw DJ, Savill NJ, et al. Estimating risk factors for farm-level transmission of disease: foot and mouth disease during the 2001 epidemic in Great Britain. Epidemics 2010;2(3):109–15.

37. Bessell PR, Shaw DJ, Savill NJ, et al. Statistical modeling of holding level susceptibility to infection during the 2001 foot and mouth disease epidemic in Great Britain. Int J Infect Dis 2010;14(3):e210–5.
38. Beck-Johnson LM, Gorsich EE, Hallman C, et al. An exploration of within-herd dynamics of a transboundary livestock disease: A foot and mouth disease case study. Epidemics 2023;42:100668.
39. Allepuz A, Stevenson M, Kivaria F, et al. Risk factors for foot-and-mouth disease in Tanzania, 2001-2006. Transbound Emerg Dis 2015;62(2):127–36.
40. Munsey A, Mwiine FN, Ochwo S, et al. Spatial distribution and risk factors for foot and mouth disease virus in Uganda: Opportunities for strategic surveillance. Prev Vet Med 2019;171:104766.
41. Perez AM, Ward MP, Carpenter TE. Epidemiological investigations of the 2001 foot-and-mouth disease outbreak in Argentina. Vet Rec 2004;154(25):777–82.
42. Mansley LM, Dunlop PJ, Whiteside SM, et al. Early dissemination of foot-and-mouth disease virus through sheep marketing in February 2001. Vet Rec 2003; 153(2):43–50.
43. Carpenter TE, O'Brien JM, Hagerman AD, et al. Epidemic and economic impacts of delayed detection of foot-and-mouth disease: a case study of a simulated outbreak in California. J Vet Diagn Invest 2011;23(1):26–33.
44. Smith MR, Sanderson MW. Modeled impacts of rapid and accurate cattle tracing in a Foot-and-Mouth Disease outbreak in the US. Prev Vet Med 2023;215:105911.
45. Bickett-Weddle DA, Sanderson MW, Parker EJ. Foreign Animal Disease Outbreaks. Vet Clin North Am Food Anim Pract 2018;34(2):341–54.
46. USDA APHIS FMD Response Plan, The red book, 2020, USDA APHIS, Veterinary Services National Center for Animal Health Emergency Management. Available at: https://www.aphis.usda.gov/animal_health/emergency_management/downloads/fmd_responseplan.pdf.
47. Supply SB. Secure beef supply. 2023. Available at: www.securebeef.org. [Accessed 10 April 2023].
48. Newman JF, Rowlands DJ, Brown F. A physico-chemical sub-grouping of the mammalian picornaviruses. J Gen Virol 1973;18(2):171–80.
49. USDA-APHIS. Disinfectants approved for use against foot-and-mouth disease virus in farm settings. 2020. Available at: https://www.aphis.usda.gov/animal_health/emergency_management/downloads/fmd-virus-disinfectants.pdf. [Accessed 12 January 2023].
50. Brown E, Nelson N, Gubbins S, et al. Environmental and air sampling are efficient methods for the detection and quantification of foot-and-mouth disease virus. J Virol Methods 2021;287:113988.
51. Colenutt C, Brown E, Nelson N, et al. Environmental Sampling as a Low-Technology Method for Surveillance of Foot-and-Mouth Disease Virus in an Area of Endemicity. Appl Environ Microbiol 2018;(16):84.
52. Mielke SR, Garabed R. Environmental persistence of foot-and-mouth disease virus applied to endemic regions. Transbound Emerg Dis 2020;67(2):543–54.
53. Stenfeldt C, Bertram MR, Smoliga GR, et al. Duration of Contagion of Foot-And-Mouth Disease Virus in Infected Live Pigs and Carcasses. Front Vet Sci 2020; 7:334.
54. Hunnam J, Duff K, Wingett M, et al. Effect of carcase decomposition on the inactivation of foot-and-mouth disease virus under northern Australian conditions. Aust Vet J 2018;96(9):332–40.
55. WOAH. Infection with foot-and-mouth disease virus. In: WOAH, ed. Terrestrial animal Health code. 2023:chap 8.8. Available at: https://www.woah.org/en/what-we-

do/standards/codes-and-manuals/terrestrial-code-online-access/?id=169&L=1&htmfile=chapitre_fmd.htm.

56. Barnett PV, Geale DW, Clarke G, et al. A Review of OIE Country Status Recovery Using Vaccinate-to-Live Versus Vaccinate-to-Die Foot-and-Mouth Disease Response Policies I: Benefits of Higher Potency Vaccines and Associated NSP DIVA Test Systems in Post-Outbreak Surveillance. Transbound Emerg Dis 2015; 62(4):367–87.

57. Hutber AM, Kitching RP, Fishwick JC, et al. Foot-and-mouth disease: the question of implementing vaccinal control during an epidemic. Vet J 2011;188(1):18–23.

58. Leforban Y, Gerbier G. Review of the status of foot and mouth disease and approach to control/eradication in Europe and Central Asia. Rev Sci Tech 2002;21(3):477–92.

59. Saraiva V. Vaccines and foot-and-mouth disease eradication in South America. Dev Biol (Basel) 2003;114:67–77.

60. Muroga N, Hayama Y, Yamamoto T, et al. The 2010 foot-and-mouth disease epidemic in Japan. J Vet Med Sci 2012;74(4):399–404.

61. Park JH, Lee KN, Ko YJ, et al. Control of foot-and-mouth disease during 2010-2011 epidemic, South Korea. Emerg Infect Dis 2013;19(4):655–9.

62. Diaz-San Segundo F, Medina GN, Stenfeldt C, et al. Foot-and-mouth disease vaccines. Vet Microbiol 2017;206:102–12.

63. USDA. NAHEMS. Guidelines: vaccination for contagious disease appendix A: FMD. 2015. Available at: https://www.cfsph.iastate.edu/pdf/fad-prep-nahems-appendix-a-vaccination-for-foot-and-mouth-disease.

64. USDA. FAD. PReP Strategy document classification of phases and types of a foot-and-mouth disease outbreak response. 2013. Available at: https://www.cfsph.iastate.edu/pdf/phases-and-types-of-an-fmd-outbreak.

65. Walz E, Evanson J, Sampedro F, et al. Planning "Plan B": The Case of Moving Cattle From an Infected Feedlot Premises During a Hypothetical Widespread FMD Outbreak in the United States. Perspective. Front Vet Sci 2020;(484):6.

66. Walz E, Middleton J, Sampedro F, et al. Modeling the Transmission of Foot and Mouth Disease to Inform Transportation of Infected Carcasses to a Disposal Site During an Outbreak Event. Original Research. Front Vet Sci 2020;(501):6.

67. McReynolds SW, Sanderson MW. Feasibility of depopulation of a large feedlot during a foot-and-mouth disease outbreak. J Am Vet Med Assoc 2014;244(3): 291–8.

68. Yadav S, Delgado AH, Hagerman AD, et al. Epidemiologic and economic considerations regarding persistently infected cattle during vaccinate-to-live strategies for control of foot-and-mouth disease in FMD-free regions. Front Vet Sci 2022;9: 1026592.

69. Hayer SS, VanderWaal K, Ranjan R, et al. Foot-and-mouth disease virus transmission dynamics and persistence in a herd of vaccinated dairy cattle in India. Transbound Emerg Dis 2018;65(2):e404–15.

Disease Investigations & Initial Response

Considerations from Policy to Farm

Kelli Kirtley Werling, DVM[a],*, Kyle Shipman, DVM[a],
Nick Lyons, MA, VetMB, MSc, PhD, MRCVS[b]

KEYWORDS

- Disease investigation • Response policies • Epidemiologic investigation
- Vaccination strategies

KEY POINTS

- Transboundary animal disease (TAD) investigations are routinely conducted to rule out diseases that are of significant economic, trade, and/or food security importance in cattle and bison.
- TAD investigations begin with notification of a suspect case to a regulatory animal health official and are followed by sample collection and submission for laboratory confirmation.
- Regulatory animal health officials, veterinary practitioners, and cattle and bison producers all play specific roles in TAD investigations.
- Regulatory officials use the findings from epidemiologic investigations to inform decision-making related to disease response policies and strategies.
- Successful implementation of disease response, with or without vaccination, requires a collaborative effort between regulatory officials, industry groups, private practitioners, and producers.

BACKGROUND

Transboundary animal disease (TAD) investigations are conducted to rule out diseases that are of significant economic, trade, and/or food security importance. State and federal animal health officials conduct these investigations in the background across the United States every day. In the past 2 decades, there have been over 21,800 investigations conducted to rule out transboundary animal diseases throughout the United States, averaging from a low of less than 1 investigation per day in 2008 to a high of 7 investigations per day in 2021[1] (**Fig. 1**).

[a] Indiana State Board of Animal Health, 1202 East 38th Street, Discovery Hall – Suite 100, Indianapolis, IN 46205, USA; [b] Animal and Plant Health Agency (APHA), Strathearn House, Broxden Business Park, Lamberkine Drive, Perth PH1 1RX, UK
* Corresponding author.
E-mail address: kwerling@boah.in.gov

Vet Clin Food Anim 40 (2024) 205–218
https://doi.org/10.1016/j.cvfa.2024.01.010
0749-0720/24/© 2024 Elsevier Inc. All rights reserved.

In 2021 alone, there were 2716 TAD investigations conducted in 46 states, the US Virgin Islands, and Puerto Rico.[1] One thousand, seven hundred fifty-four of these investigations were vesicular complaints of which 83 were in bovids[1] (**Fig. 2**).

This article will focus on TAD investigations,[2,3] initial response activities,[4] vaccination strategies, and role-specific considerations, all based on known international standards as defined by the World Organisation for Animal Health (WOAH), founded as OIE (Office International des Epizooties).

DISCUSSION
Notification of Suspected Transboundary Animal Disease and Initiating Transboundary Animal Disease Investigation

Notification of suspected TADs oftentimes occurs with a veterinary practitioner observing clinical signs consistent with a TAD and notifying their state animal health official (SAHO) or federal representative. Other methods of notification include a producer noticing suspicious clinical signs and contacting the SAHO directly, a public health veterinarian at a slaughter facility noticing suspicious clinical signs and contacting an animal health official, or a diagnostic laboratory testing for a TAD based on diagnostician discretion, and notifying the SAHO if test results indicate a TAD is suspected. Upon notification, it is the responsibility of the SAHO to determine if the report of a potential TAD warrants an investigation by evaluating the reported clinical signs and the producer or practitioner's overall clinical suspicion of a TAD. TAD investigations may only be initiated by a SAHO, federal animal health official, or designated officials from their offices. Regardless of the method of notification, the SAHO will coordinate with the federal animal health official to initiate an investigation.

Initiating an Investigation

Initial actions
The initial actions of a disease investigation are those that occur within the first 24 hours beginning at the time of notification. These actions include assigning a regulatory veterinarian as a foreign animal disease diagnostician (FADD), obtaining an

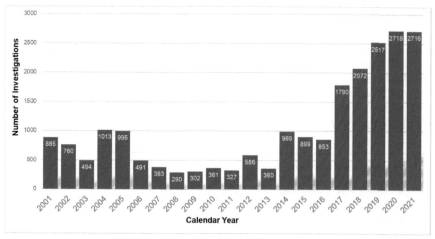

Fig. 1. U.S. transboundary animal disease (TAD) investigations from 2001 to 2021. (*From* USDA APHIS- Calendar Year 2021 update: FAD Investigation report; with permission.)

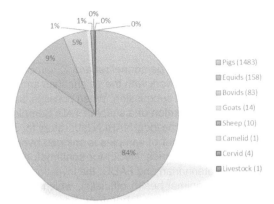

Fig. 2. 2021 US TAD investigations involving vesicular lesions, by species. (*From* USDA APHIS-Calendar Year 2021 update: FAD Investigation report; with permission.)

investigation referral control number from the federal animal health official, performing an initial epidemiologic investigation, and completing a field investigation.[2,3]

Assigning a foreign animal disease diagnostician to a disease investigation
The SAHO will assign the most readily available FADD to complete an investigation; however, if an FADD is not available, the most qualified person can be dispatched, who could be the licensed and accredited veterinary practitioner who reported the potential TAD or who has a veterinarian-client-patient-relationship (VCPR) with the producer who reported the suspected TAD. In this instance, the veterinary practitioner will be authorized to collect samples on behalf of the SAHO; however, an FADD will be assigned to provide guidance but may not be the individual dispatched to the site during these initial actions. The FADD will work closely with the private veterinarian and the producer throughout the entire investigation process.

Investigation communications
The FADD will contact the veterinarian or producer who reported the suspicion of disease and coordinate a field investigation. Oftentimes, the veterinarian who reported the disease suspicion will serve as the communication liaison between the producer and FADD. Designating a primary point of contact for communication between all parties involved ensures clarity of communication and prevents accidental misinformation. Public information will be disseminated in coordination between the SAHO and the federal animal health authorities upon disease confirmation.

Hold orders and quarantines
The FADD, on behalf of the SAHO, may place a verbal hold order or written quarantine on the affected location while the investigation is ongoing. The attitudes and willingness to cooperate of the producer, along with the clinical suspicion of the veterinarian, and the prevalence of clinical signs are all considerations that are explored to help determine if a verbal hold order or a written quarantine is placed. If either restriction is put in place, movements of animals or animal products are prohibited until released at the discretion of the SAHO. A preliminary test result from the National Animal Health Laboratory Network (NAHLN) laboratory, which is a USDA-approved cooperating state or university animal disease diagnostic laboratory, may be sufficient for the sending and receiving SAHOs to allow movement to resume with all parties agreeing to the movement. Preliminary results are generally returned within 24 hours, whereas

confirmatory results may take 4 to 6 days, depending on the sample priority classification (see later section).

Collection and shipment of samples

The FADD will consult with laboratory personnel regarding sample collection, preparation, and handling.[2] The FADD will work with the veterinarian and/or producer at the site to collect samples for diagnostic submission. When possible, sample collection is completed within 24 hours of notification of a suspect TAD. Samples are collected in duplicate with one set being sent to the local NAHLN laboratory for same-day or overnight preliminary testing. The other set of samples is shipped overnight to 1 of the 2 National Veterinary Services Laboratories (NVSL) for confirmatory testing. Based on the clinical suspicion of the veterinarian and FADD, the investigation will be classified by the SAHO and the federal animal health official(s), which will determine priority placed on sample processing through the laboratory. Samples of higher priority (ie, higher clinical suspicion of a TAD) will be expedited through this entire process. Sending samples to the local NAHLN lab is optional, but it has been found to facilitate preliminary decision-making in the interim while waiting for confirmatory test results.

If the veterinary practitioner who reported the disease was assigned as the FADD, they are authorized to collect samples on behalf of the SAHO. Chain of custody of the samples is maintained throughout the collection and shipping process by the FADD. Considerations of the SAHO in determining if a private practitioner should collect samples for a suspected TAD include

- Private practitioner is already onsite and willing to collect samples on behalf of the regulatory official. This prioritizes biosecurity while limiting the impact of potential exposure of personnel.
- A state or federal FADD is not available or will be delayed, and the private practitioner is licensed and accredited.
- The private practitioner has all the necessary materials and supplies for sample collection, including the correct transport media.

The veterinary practitioner should be careful to follow strict biosecurity measures and refrain from contact with other susceptible animal species until test results are received. Recommended biosecurity measures include

- Disinfect all non-disposable supplies and equipment. Consider leaving these supplies on site and returning for them later following a lifting of restrictions.
- Dispose of all single-use materials on site.
- Wash and sanitize hands and footwear before leaving the site.
- Clean and disinfect high touchpoint areas of the vehicle. Internally, focus on the steering wheel, shift mechanism, and floorboard. On the exterior, focus on running boards, wheels, wheel wells, undercarriage, and any surface that made direct contact with contaminated materials.
- Shower and launder clothing prior to resuming normal activities.

Epidemiologic Investigation

The FADD will initiate an epidemiologic investigation and gather information pertinent to the case in coordination with the veterinary practitioner. Information can be collected via various methodologies to provide flexibility and ensure enhanced biosecurity measures are observed. It is important that an initial case history is prepared promptly, and the FADD transmits it to all parties involved in the investigation as soon as possible. Pertinent information to consider in the case history includes

- Date and time of initial report,
- Contact information for the individual making the report,
- Primary clinical complaints and/or suspected disease agent,
- Number of animals and species on premises,
- Number of animals and species affected,
- Duration of illness or clinical signs observed,
- History of animal and/or animal product movement on and off the premises,
- History of international travel.

Following disease confirmation, the regulatory FADD will conduct a more in-depth epidemiologic investigation. For foot-and-mouth disease (FMD), this includes investigating suspected disease introduction by aging vesicular lesions if present. The correlation between viral introduction, viral shedding, and lesion progression further informs contact tracing, response activities, and/or vaccination strategies.

Transmission timelines—the case of foot-and-mouth disease

Timelines are an essential tool in the investigation of disease outbreaks. Tracing windows are created to assist in the identification of possible sources of infection using knowledge of the onset of clinical signs (typically defined as "day 0" in the timeline), the incubation period (the time from infection to onset of clinical signs), and the infectious period (the time during which an individual animal may transmit infection to another susceptible host) (**Fig. 3**).

In the case of FMD, the creation of timelines can be informed by lesion aging to help establish the onset of clinical signs and the tracing windows (**Fig. 4**). At the epidemiologic unit level, it is important to find and estimate the age of the oldest lesion which will include identifying and examining all epidemiologic groups. It may not be feasible to examine all individual animals; therefore, clinical judgment of which animals to examine may need to be applied. The prevalence of lesion ages in different groups may assist with the wider epidemiologic investigation.

Lesion aging

Under field conditions in live animals, oral lesions are typically used for lesion aging as feet can be more difficult to examine and are commonly complicated by the presence of secondary bacterial infections. Within the oral cavity, lesions are typically observed on the dental pad, dorsal aspect of the apical tongue, and oral vestibule. Lesions are occasionally observed on the external nose area or around the edges of the lips. Examination should be systematic to ensure all areas are evaluated to minimize the possibility of missing lesions. Care must be taken to not assume lesions present in the lingual fossa are due to FMD, as these are often observed in non-affected cattle, presumably related to the type of forage being consumed.

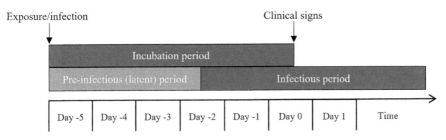

e.g., five-day incubation period, infectious from two days prior to onset of clinical signs

Fig. 3. Foot-and-mouth disease (FMD) exposure to clinical signs timeline.

Day	Date	Source Window	Spread Window
-14	August 13th		
-13	August 14th		
-12	August 15th		
-11	August 16th		
-10	August 17th		
-9	August 18th		
-8	August 19th		
-7	August 20th		
-6	August 21st		
-5	August 22nd		
-4	August 23rd		
-3	August 24th		
-2	August 25th		
-1	August 26th		
0	August 27th		
1	August 28th		
2	August 29th		
3	August 30th		
4	August 31st		
5	September 1st		

Example timeline for a FMD outbreak investigation, with the oldest lesion in the herd estimated as 4-5 days with other animals in the herd having newer lesions. For this timeline, the incubation period is assumed to be between 1 and 14 days, but most likely 2-6 days prior to the onset of clinical signs. Onward transmission is assumed to start 2 days prior to the onset of clinical signs but is high risk from day 0 onwards. In the figure, green indicates relatively lower risk, while red is the higher risk period.

Fig. 4. FMD transmission as determined by lesion aging.

When establishing the ages of lesions, the following are considered:[5,6]

- Presence of intact fluid-filled vesicles and epithelial flaps.
- Color—Lesions are initially red and become pink and then gray over time with advancing epithelization and scarring.
- Edges—Margins are initially rough or sharp, becoming rounded over time.
- Fibrin—Similar in appearance to epithelium but is typically yellow in color and more homogenous. This distinction is important for both lesion aging and diagnostic purposes.

A variety of lesion ages can be observed in an individual animal; therefore, it is important to establish the oldest lesion at this level. Lesion aging is approximate and there is greater uncertainty with advancing lesion age. Generally, when lesions are older than 2 days, it is advisable to consider a range of dates rather than a specific number of days. The oldest date within the estimated range should be used to inform timelines to give a more conservative approximation of the tracing windows. It is also recommended to supplement the lesion age with additional clinical information (eg, drop in milk production, decreased feed intake), particularly with older lesion ages and the associated uncertainty.

Once the date of onset of clinical signs (day 0) has been estimated, the tracing windows can be defined. When determining the source, the oldest observed lesion in the epidemiologic unit is used. Newer lesions and associated clinical signs allow for the determination of disease spread within a herd which may be further informed by serologic investigations.

Tracings are identified based on observations, records, and interviews. Tracings should be prioritized based on the high-risk periods for source and spread (see **Fig. 4**) and the type of movement identified (for example, tracing movement of live animals may take precedence over tracing movements of people). This prioritization is critical in the face of many outbreaks with limited resources.

Subsequent Actions

Waiting for test results
While waiting for confirmatory test results, documentation of all the actions taken to this point in the investigation must be compiled and entered into the database of record. Follow-up communications between all parties occur during this time. The FADD will perform regular check-ins to ensure that morbidity and mortality in the herd is not changing/increasing as well as checking in on the mental and emotional health of the veterinarian and producer. Local mental health resources can be provided as needed. Those experiencing mental distress or suicidal crisis can call or text the National Suicide and Crisis Lifeline at 9-8-8 for confidential support 24/7.

Case closure
Upon receipt of negative confirmatory test results from NVSL, a verbal hold order or written quarantine can be released, and all restrictions lifted. Upon confirmation of a TAD from NVSL, a response is initiated. Disease response is not the focus of this article; however, some global policy considerations as they relate to initial response activities are included. If an investigation identifies a TAD, immediate response considerations that may be implemented on-farm based on global policy include assignment of control areas and considerations for vaccination.[4]

Control areas
A critical component of a TAD response is the designation of zones and areas, and classification of premises for use in movement and disease control efforts. These definitions are conserved across most of the TADs; however, for purposes of this discussion, we will focus on FMD response. For FMD, the perimeter of the control area should be at least 10 km (~6.21 miles) beyond the perimeter of the infected premises.[4] The size of the control area depends on the circumstances of the outbreak and can be modified or redefined as epidemiologic information becomes available. The **Tables 1–3** summarize the various premises designations and geographic zones used during a disease response. **Fig. 5** provides a geospatial illustration of these response zones and areas.

Response activities vary considerably depending on premises classification and zone designation. Major activities for infected premises include depopulation, disposal, and pathogen elimination, or implementation of a vaccination strategy. Major activities

Table 1
Summary of premises designations[4]

Premises	Definition
Infected Premises (IP)	Premises where presumptive positive case or confirmed positive case exists based on laboratory results, compatible clinical signs, foot-and-mouth disease (FMD) case definition, and international standards.
Contact Premises (CP)	Premises with susceptible animals that may have been exposed to FMD, either directly or indirectly, including but not limited to exposure to animals, animal products, fomites, or people from Infected Premises.
Suspect Premises (SP)	Premises under investigation due to the presence of susceptible animals reported to have clinical signs compatible with FMD. This is intended to be a short-term premises designation.
At-Risk Premises (ARP)	Premises that have susceptible animals, but none of those susceptible animals have clinical signs compatible with FMD. Premises objectively demonstrate that it is not an Infected Premises, Contact Premises, or Suspect Premises. At-Risk Premises seek to move susceptible animals or products within the Control Area by permit. Only At-Risk Premises are eligible to become Monitored Premises.
Monitored Premises (MP)	Premises objectively demonstrate that it is not Infected Premises, Contact Premises, or Suspect Premises. Only At-Risk Premises are eligible to become Monitored Premises. Monitored Premises meet a set of defined criteria in seeking to move susceptible animals or products out of the Control Area by permit.
Free Premises (FP)	Premises outside of a Control Area and not a Contact or Suspect Premises.
Vaccinated Premises (VP)	Premises where emergency vaccination has been performed. This may be a secondary premises designation.

Adapted from USDA Foot-and-Mouth Disease Response Plan: The Red Book ~ 2020; with permission.

for non-infected premises include disease surveillance and movement controls established to move susceptible animals or products within, into, or out of a Control Area. The **Table 3** summarizes these activities.

Surveillance activities may differ from the aforementioned activities if vaccination strategies are utilized. While regulatory veterinarians may perform some of the initial surveillance activities, it is likely that the veterinary practitioner and/or their designee(s) may be called upon to assist with vaccination of animals and collection of diagnostic samples for surveillance activities as the disease response continues.

Vaccination Strategies

Availability
Of the major TADs of cattle and bison, vaccines are potentially available for contagious bovine pleuropneumonia, FMD, lumpy skin disease, and rift valley fever. The case of FMD vaccination deserves special mention due to its potential use in the United States in the event of an incursion and the considerations required for decision-making.

FMD is endemic in large parts of Africa and Asia and some parts of South America, and vaccination is used on a large scale in its control and the maintenance of some disease-free zones.[7] The properties of FMD vaccines have been extensively reviewed elsewhere,[8–10] but the majority in use today are killed/inactivated and contain aqueous

Table 2 Minimum sizes of areas and zones[4]	
Zone or Area	**Minimum Size and Details**
Infected Zone (IZ)	Zone that immediately surrounds an Infected Premises. Perimeter should be at least 3 km (1.86 miles) beyond perimeters of presumptive or confirmed Infected Premises. Will depend on disease agent and epidemiologic circumstances. This zone may be redefined as the outbreak continues.
Buffer Zone (BZ)	Zone that immediately surrounds an Infected Zone or a Contact Premises. Perimeter should be at least 7 km (4.35 miles) beyond the perimeter of the Infected Zone. Width is generally not less than the minimum radius of the associated Infected Zone but may be much larger. This zone may be redefined as the outbreak continues.
Control Area (CA)	Consists of an Infected Zone and a Buffer Zone. Perimeter should be at least 10 km (6.21 miles) beyond the perimeter of the closest Infected Premises. Please see Tables 4–7[4] for factors that influence the size of the Control Area. This area may be redefined as the outbreak continues.
Surveillance Zone (SZ)	Zone outside and along the border of a Control Area. Width should be at least 10 km (6.21 miles) but may be much larger.

Adapted from USDA Foot-and-Mouth Disease Response Plan: The Red Book – 2020; with permission.

Table 3 Response activities summary[4]	
Premises, Zone or Area	**Response Activities**
Suspect Premises (SP)	Immediately investigate and sample. Consider repeating every other day through a full incubation period if initial test results are negative.
Contact Premises (CP)	Sample every 5 d for 14 d. Optimum frequency depends on incubation period and exposure risk.
Control Area (CA)	At-Risk Premises (ARP)—Sample every 10 d until 56 d after the last detected case. Optimum frequency depends on incubation period and exposure risk. Must meet a set of defined criteria in seeking to move susceptible animals or products within, into, or out of the Control Area by permit. Monitored Premises (MP)—Sample every 10 d until 56 d after the last detected case, or more frequently as required for movement testing. Testing should occur for a minimum of 5 times for the duration of the quarantine. Optimum frequency depends on incubation period and exposure risk. Must meet a set of defined criteria in seeking to move susceptible animals or products within, into, or out of the Control Area by permit.
Surveillance Zone (SZ)	Surveillance testing once to confirm lack of spread and repeated every 21 d until 56 d after the last detected case. Or consider repeating 2–3 times prior to release of the control area.

Adapted from USDA Foot-and-Mouth Disease Response Plan: The Red Book – 2020; with permission.

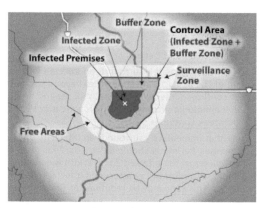

Fig. 5. Example of response zones and areas. (USDA Foot-and-mouth disease response plan; The Red Book 2020; with permission.)

or oil-based adjuvants. An adenovirus-vectored FMD vaccine is also licensed in the United States.

Foot-and-mouth disease vaccine properties

A critical consideration and limitation of FMD vaccines is that there is no cross-protection between serotypes and protection is variable for strains within a serotype. A key property of many modern FMD vaccines is the removal of the non-immunogenic non-structural proteins (NSP) which allows the use of tests that differentiate infected from vaccinated animals (DIVA) tests. Animals that have been vaccinated with an NSP-purified vaccine will not seroconvert to NSP unless they have been exposed to infection. Sero-surveillance is an important tool for the demonstration of freedom from infection in vaccinated populations.[11] The WOAH Terrestrial Code allows for countries or zones to have free status with or without vaccination, although the latter is more desirable from a trade perspective.[12,13]

Considerations for use of foot-and-mouth disease vaccination

Vaccination may also be used in response to a viral incursion into an FMD-free country or zone, with numerous countries electing to do so.[14–16] Vaccination may reduce the scale of the epidemic, which can in turn reduce the need for stamping-out (ie, the killing and disposal of confirmed or suspected infected animals and those that are likely to have been exposed) and therefore, the negative impacts of stamping out on the food supply and the environment. Through slowing the outbreak, vaccination may also allow more effective allocation of limited resources that are likely to be severely stretched with an FMD incursion. The decision on whether to use vaccination in response to FMD detection (known as emergency or reactive vaccination) is challenging and complex, with considerations including the characteristics of the epidemic, the likelihood of a non-vaccination strategy to be successful, and the feasibility of delivering an effective vaccination policy. **Fig. 6** provides an overview of traditional FMD response strategies with and without the use of vaccination.[4]

Another critical consideration is the impact on international trade and the time it takes to regain WOAH FMD-free status. A country or zone may recover FMD-free status 3 months after the slaughter and disposal of the last animal when a stamping-out policy is used, subject to adequate surveillance to demonstrate freedom. When vaccination is used, stamping out must include all vaccinated animals (ie, "vaccination-to-kill" or

Strategy or Strategies	Definition of Strategy	Likelihood of Use	Example of Application
Stamping-Out (No Emergency Vaccination)	Depopulation of clinically affected and in-contact susceptible animals.	Possible (if outbreak is contained in jurisdictional areas in which FMD can be readily contained and further dissemination of the virus is unlikely).	Stamping-out Infected Premises.
Stamping-Out Modified with Emergency Vaccination to Kill	Depopulation of clinically affected and in-contact susceptible animals and vaccination of at-risk animals, with subsequent depopulation and disposal of vaccinated animals. Depopulation and disposal of vaccinated animals may be delayed until logistically feasible.	Possible (if outbreak is contained in jurisdictional areas in which FMD can be readily contained and further dissemination of the virus is unlikely).	Stamping-out Infected Premises, emergency vaccination to kill within the selected areas of the Buffer Zone in Containment Vaccination Zones.
Stamping-Out Modified with Emergency Vaccination to Slaughter	Depopulation of clinically affected and in-contact susceptible animals and vaccination of at-risk animals, with subsequent slaughter of vaccinated animals if animals are eligible for slaughter under USDA FSIS and/or State and Tribal authority and rules.	Highly likely (depending on the type of the FMD outbreak).	Stamping-out Infected Premises; emergency vaccination to slaughter within the Control Area in Containment Vaccination Zones.
Stamping-Out Modified with Emergency Vaccination to Live	Depopulation of clinically affected and in-contact susceptible animals and vaccination of at-risk animals, without subsequent depopulation of vaccinated animals. Vaccinated animals intended for breeding, slaughter, or other purposes live out their useful lives.	Highly likely (depending on the type of the FMD outbreak).	Stamping-out Infected Premises; emergency vaccination to live outside of the Control Area in Protection Vaccination Zones.
Combination of Stamping-Out Modified with Emergency Vaccination to Kill, Slaughter, and Live	Combination of emergency vaccination to kill, slaughter, and live.	Highly likely (depending on the type of the FMD outbreak).	Stamping-out Infected Premises; emergency vaccination to slaughter within the Control Area in Containment Vaccination Zones and emergency vaccination to live outside.
Vaccination to Live (without Stamping-Out)	Vaccination used without depopulation of infected animals or subsequent depopulation or slaughter of vaccinated animals.	Less likely (unlikely to be implemented at start of outbreak).	No stamping-out Infected Premises; Vaccination to live outside of the Control Area in Protection Vaccination Zones.
No Action	FMD would take its course in the affected population; other measures may be implemented to control and contain FMD spread.	Unlikely in domestic animals.	Quarantine and movement control measures; biosecurity measures; cleaning and disinfection measures implemented. No stamping-out and no vaccination.

Fig. 6. Overview of traditional foot-and-mouth disease response strategies. (USDA Foot-and-mouth disease response plan; The Red Book 2020; with permission.)

"vaccination-to-die"). However, if vaccinated animals are not killed ("vaccination-to-live"), the period is extended to 6 months after the last affected animal is depopulated or the last vaccination is administered, coupled with NSP sero-surveillance necessary to support the application for FMD-free status.[17,18] A case has been made that these waiting times should be equivalent given advances in epidemiology, diagnostics, and vaccines.[15]

If a country elects to use vaccination, the strategy will be determined by the particular epidemic and the feasibility of delivery. If the epidemic is widespread, vaccination may be considered over a large geographic area. If outbreaks are more contained, use might be considered at a smaller scale covering herds in the areas surrounding individual affected premises or outbreak clusters. The current US policy on vaccination acknowledges that stamping-out alone is unlikely to be viable except for a "very small, focal outbreak," and an FMD outbreak typology has been proposed to guide decision-making on the use of vaccination.[19]

Successful implementation

An emergency or reactive FMD vaccination campaign is more likely to be successful when the following key components are included.

- High antigen payload (with a vaccine potency in excess of 6 PD_{50})[20]
- Close "match" between the circulating strain and the vaccine strain[20]
- High vaccine application aiming to vaccinate all FMD-susceptible species
- Rapid deployment
- Rigorous active surveillance to determine the location of infected animals or herds
- Strict movement restrictions

Vaccine banks

Vaccine banks store strategic reserves of concentrated antigen for rapid vaccine deployment. These can be rapidly formulated with a delivery of deployable vaccine 10 to 14 days following an order being placed.[19] The selection of strains to include in these banks relies upon effective global surveillance to understand the geographic distributions of different strains and an understanding of the effectiveness of vaccines in use. A recent publication has outlined a novel Prioritization of Antigen Management with International Surveillance Tool (PRAGMATIST) to assist bank managers with strain selection according to their region of interest.[21] The United States has access to 2 FMD vaccine banks, one that is shared with Canada and Mexico (the North American Foot and Mouth Disease Vaccine Bank [NAFMDVB]) and another for exclusive use by the United States available since 2020 (the National Animal Vaccine and Veterinary Countermeasures Bank [NAVVCB] or "National Bank"). For the latter, the aim is to "acquire 10 to 25 million doses of each of the 10 to 12 highest risk strains of FMD."[19] Similarly to the "National Bank," Canada plans to create an FMD vaccine bank for their exclusive use. The NAFMDVB also participates in an agreement including the Australian and New Zealand FMD vaccine banks which supports access to additional vaccines in the event of an FMD outbreak in any of the 5 participating countries. However, despite the potential availability of these vaccines, in the event of a "widespread" or "catastrophic" FMD outbreak, it is acknowledged that vaccine supply will be unable to meet the demand.[19]

SUMMARY

TAD investigations are conducted routinely across the United States to rule out diseases of significant economic, trade, and/or food security importance. Established protocols exist for TAD investigations and disease response based on national and international policy; however, now more than ever, private practitioners may be called upon to assist in these investigations and response activities and may play an important role in communications, sample collection, and disease surveillance. Regulatory officials use the findings from epidemiologic investigations to inform decision-making related to disease response policies and strategies. Successful implementation of disease response, with or without vaccination, requires a collaborative effort between regulatory officials, industry groups, private practitioners, and producers. The more informed and collaborative private veterinarians, producers, and regulatory animal health officials are, the better able they will be to prevent TAD disease introduction and maintain healthy, viable herds for a thriving agricultural economy.

CLINICS CARE POINTS

- Become familiar with the clinical signs associated with TADs in cattle or bison.
- Call your state or federal animal health official if you suspect a TAD.
- TAD investigations begin with notification of a suspect case to a regulatory animal health official and are followed by sample collection and submission for laboratory confirmation.
- Be prepared to assist regulatory animal health officials during a TAD investigation by serving as a communication liaison and/or performing sample collection.

ACKNOWLEDGMENTS

The authors would like to acknowledge and thank the United States Department of Agriculture for use of the materials on the Foreign Animal Disease Preparedness and Response Plan (FAD PReP) website and acknowledge the subject matter expertise of the European Commission for the Control of Foot-and-Mouth Disease (EuFMD).

DISCLOSURE

K. Shipman and K.K. Werling are employed by the Indiana State Board of Animal Health. N. Lyons is employed by the Animal and Plant Health Agency. The authors have nothing additional to disclose.

REFERENCES

1. USDA APHIS VS, Calendar Year 2021 Update: FAD Investigation Report, Available at: https://www.aphis.usda.gov/animal_health/emergency_management/downloads/summary-fad-investigations-cy2021.pdf. (Accessed 8 August 2023).
2. USDA APHIS VS. Foreign Animal Disease Investigation Manual (FAD PReP Manual 4.0). 2022. Available at: https://www.usdatraining.com/powerpoint_docs/FADD_Manual_digital.pdf. [Accessed 8 August 2023].
3. USDA APHIS VS. VS Guidance 12001.4: Policy for the Investigation of Potential Foreign Animal Disease/Emerging Disease Incidents (FAD/EDI). 2020. Available at: https://www.aphis.usda.gov/animal_health/lab_info_services/downloads/VSG_12001.pdf. [Accessed 8 August 2023].
4. USDA APHIS VS. Foot-and-Mouth Disease Response Plan: The Red Book. 2020. Available at: https://www.aphis.usda.gov/animal_health/emergency_management/downloads/fmd_responseplan.pdf. [Accessed 8 August 2023].
5. European Commission for the Control of Foot-and-mouth Disease. A field guide to estimating the age of Foot-and-Mouth disease lesions. Available at: https://www.fao.org/fileadmin/user_upload/eufmd/docs/training/EnglLesionageing.pdf. [Accessed 22 September 2023].
6. Department of Environment, Food and Rural Affairs. Foot and Mouth Disease Ageing of Lesions. 2005. Available at: https://usercontent.one/wp/epiwebb.se/wp-content/uploads/2018/12/DEFRA-ageing-of-lesions.pdf. [Accessed 22 September 2023].
7. World Organisation for Animal Health (OIE). Chapter 8.8 Infection with Foot and Mouth Disease Virus. In: Terrestrial Animal Health Code. Paris, France: World Organisation for Animal Health (OIE); 2015. p. 455–77.

8. Doel TR. FMD vaccines. Virus Res 2003;91:81–99.
9. Diaz-San Segundo F, Medina GN, Stenfeldt C, et al. Foot-and-mouth disease vaccines. Vet Microbiol 2017;206:102–12.
10. Belsham GJ. Towards improvements in foot-and-mouth disease vaccine performance. Acta Vet Scand 2020;62:20.
11. Paton DJ, de Clercq K, Greiner M, et al. Application of non-structural protein antibody tests in substantiating freedom from foot-and-mouth disease virus infection after emergency vaccination of cattle. Vaccine 2006;24:6503–12.
12. World Organisation for Animal Health (OIE). Chapter 8.8 Infection with Foot and Mouth Disease Virus, Article 8.8.2. In: Terrestrial Animal Health Code. Paris, France: World Organisation for Animal Health (OIE); 2015. p. 455–6.
13. World Organisation for Animal Health (OIE). Chapter 8.8 Infection with Foot and Mouth Disease Virus, Article 8.8.3. In: Terrestrial Animal Health Code. Paris, France: World Organisation for Animal Health (OIE); 2015. p. 456–7.
14. Bouma A, Elbers AR, Dekker A, et al. The foot-and-mouth disease epidemic in The Netherlands in 2001. Prev Vet Med 2003;57:155–66.
15. Muroga N, Hayama Y, Yamamoto T, et al. The 2010 foot-and-mouth disease epidemic in Japan. J Vet Med Sci 2012;74:399–404.
16. Park JH, Tark D, Lee KN, et al. Control of type O foot-and-mouth disease by vaccination in Korea, 2014-2015. J Vet Sci 2018;19:271–9.
17. World Organisation for Animal Health (OIE). Chapter 8.8 Infection with Foot and Mouth Disease Virus, Article 8.8.7. In: Terrestrial Animal Health Code. Paris, France: World Organisation for Animal Health (OIE); 2015. p. 459–60.
18. Geale DW, Barnett PV, Clarke GW, et al. A Review of OIE Country Status Recovery Using Vaccinate-to-Live Versus Vaccinate-to-Die Foot-and-Mouth Disease Response Policies II: Waiting Periods After Emergency Vaccination in FMD Free Countries. Transbound Emerg Dis 2015;62:388–406.
19. United States Department of Agriculture. Foot-and-Mouth Disease Vaccination Policy in the United States. 2020. Available at: https://www.aphis.usda.gov/animal_health/emergency_management/downloads/fmd-vac-policy.pdf. [Accessed 22 September 2023].
20. World Organisation for Animal Health (OIE). Chapter 3.1.8. Foot and Mouth Disease (infection with foot and mouth disease virus). In: Manual of Diagnostic Tests and Vaccines for Terrestrial Animals. Paris, France: World Organisation for Animal Health (OIE); 2022. p. 1–34.
21. Ludi AB, McLaws M, Armson B, et al. PRAGMATIST: A tool to prioritize foot-and-mouth disease virus antigens held in vaccine banks. Front Vet Sci 2022;9:1029075.

Readiness and Response
The Practitioner's Role

Carla L. Huston, DVM, PhD, dip. ACVPM (Epidemiology)[a,*],
John Wenzel, DVM[b,c]

KEYWORDS

- Foreign animal diseases • Disaster management • Disaster training • Biosecurity
- Veterinarians • First responder

KEY POINTS

- The threat of foreign animal diseases is steadily increasing with the ease of travel and trade of people, animals, animal products, and feedstuffs.
- Veterinary practitioners can play a vital role in a community's preparedness for, response to, and recovery from an animal disease outbreak.
- Resources are available for veterinarians to become trained in emergency management and foreign animal disease recognition and control.
- Training and exercising preparedness plans are necessary for an effective and efficient response to a foreign animal disease outbreak.
- A foreign animal disease outbreak requires whole-community involvement.

INTRODUCTION

It is likely that veterinarians will find themselves involved in assisting with a disaster at some point in their professional career. Cattle and bison are affected by many types of disasters, from accidental (or nonintentional) to intentional. Nonintentional disasters include weather-related events, such as wildfires, tornadoes, hurricanes, floods, and blizzards; or naturally occurring disease-related events, such as transboundary or foreign animal disease (FAD) outbreaks. Intentional disasters occur from the result of man-made purposeful acts, such as arson, intentional release of chemical hazards, or terrorist acts (including agroterrorism and bioterrorism).

According to the US Department of Agriculture (USDA) National Agricultural Statistics Service, there were more than 90 million cattle and calves, including more than 9.4

[a] Mississippi State University College of Veterinary Medicine, PO Box 6100, Mississippi State, MS 39762, USA; [b] Extension Animal Sciences and Natural Resources, New Mexico State University, Las Cruces, NM 88003, USA; [c] Southwest Veterinary Services, PO Box 5146, Silver City, NM 88062, USA
* Corresponding author.
E-mail address: huston@cvm.msstate.edu

Vet Clin Food Anim 40 (2024) 219–232
https://doi.org/10.1016/j.cvfa.2024.01.011
0749-0720/24/© 2024 Elsevier Inc. All rights reserved.

million dairy cattle and 30.3 million beef cows, on inventory in the United States in January 2019.[1] With these numbers of livestock, and the growing risk of FAD incursions in the United States every year because of travel and trade of people, animals, animal products, and feedstuffs, veterinarians should be prepared for the next disease-related disaster. In addition to the direct and immediate impact such a disaster can have on the people and animals in their community, an FAD can have devastating effects on the agricultural economy for years to come.[2,3] Furthermore, as evidenced following the 2001 foot-and-mouth disease (FMD) outbreak in the United Kingdom, long-term social and mental distress among the farming and nonfarming communities can occur.[4]

HISTORY AND SIGNIFICANCE

As early as 1948, veterinarians were involved in addressing the potential health effects of atomic explosions on animals, such as injuries and shock, and in establishing quarantine zones.[5] Although zoning remains an important component of hazard mitigation strategies, the role of the veterinarian has changed with the times. The USDA established the veterinary accreditation program in 1921 so private practitioners could aid in controlling animal diseases.[6] Initial accreditation training covered animal identification, documentation and certificates of veterinary inspection, diseases foreign to the United States (now termed foreign animal diseases), and other regulatory topics. Recent revisions in the veterinary accreditation process include training modules covering basic emergency management concepts and all-hazards preparation, planning, response, and recovery associated with animals in disasters.[7] The bovine tuberculosis and brucellosis eradication programs are two examples of federal response to diseases that relied heavily on the involvement of accredited veterinary practitioners.

Animals can serve as sentinels for emerging and zoonotic diseases, making veterinarians a first line of defense against public health disasters. Veterinary surveillance was instrumental in identifying the 1999 West Nile Virus incursion and the 2003 Monkeypox outbreak, which highlights the urgency of providing an all-hazards training to the veterinary practitioner. Due in part to the wide devastation and immense media coverage following the 2001 FMD outbreak in the United Kingdom, much emphasis is now being placed on the preparedness against an FAD incursion into the United States. The threat of any disease that could have such an immense and global financial impact, when intentionally introduced, would also be considered a bioterrorist or agroterrorist event with enormous consequences.[8]

Although the 2001 FMD outbreak in the United Kingdom had an estimated impact between $12 and 18 billion, studies of the economic cost of a modern day incursion into the United States have reached $228 billion.[8] The economic impacts would come from lost international trade and disrupted interstate trade, and from costs directly associated with the eradication effort, such as depopulation, disposal, cleaning and disinfection, and indemnity. Indirect costs may include loss of income or employment, loss of production, loss of market, and loss of related businesses. Long-term economic effects of an FAD can potentially result from reallocation of land utilization and decreases in rural community development.[9]

Veterinarians have the knowledge and skills to assist in preparedness, response, and recovery activities surrounding animal disasters, and veterinarians in the United States and Canada have been encouraged to take leadership roles in local, state, and federal efforts.[10,11] Since 1984, many disaster-related organizations have actively incorporated animal interests into their response plans.[12] Over the years, veterinarians have had many opportunities to participate in disaster management through various national agencies including the USDA National Animal Health Emergency Response Corps, the American Veterinary Medical Foundation Veterinary Medical Assistance Teams, and the Department of Health and Human Services National Veterinary Response Teams. These agencies have been instrumental in the response to and recovery from many national disasters, including multiple hurricanes, animal disease outbreaks, such as highly pathogenic avian influenza, and the Deepwater Horizon oil spill, which challenged veterinarians to use their knowledge of hazardous materials and personal protective equipment (PPE).[13]

Because of the nature of disaster occurrences and potential for long-term recovery, state and local jurisdictions have been encouraged to form state animal response teams (SARTs) and local or community emergency response teams. However, the formation and use of these resources remains highly variable across the United States.[14] Potential roles for practitioners are found by contacting the local/state emergency management agency or the local emergency planning committee. Local emergency planning committees are usually comprised of various community members, in addition to first responders and emergency management directors. Opportunities for veterinary involvement may also be available at the national level with private or nongovernmental agencies, such as the American Red Cross; however, in the case of an FAD, state and federal animal health officials have jurisdiction and oversee any and all responding entities.

CHALLENGES

Clearly, there is a need for veterinary practitioners to be trained in readiness and response to an FAD outbreak. However, there are many challenges that they may face in their efforts to become competent disaster managers in the face of an FAD. Historically, disaster management training has not been included in the veterinary curriculum, similar to the situation with physicians, who receive little to no formal training in disaster preparedness and response.[15] Veterinary curricula are faced with time limits in the traditional curriculum, making substantial change, such as the addition of disaster management training, difficult. Furthermore, there is limited availability of experienced responders to train the next generation of veterinarians. Diseases considered FADs are not found in the United States, so experience in the detection and control of such diseases is limited in US-trained veterinarians. Training has been largely limited to textbook information, disease scenario simulations, or exercises completed in initial veterinary school training and USDA accreditation.

Similarly, busy practitioners, exasperated by the shortage of veterinary practitioners in rural communities, are limited in time available to devote to activities like disaster preparedness and response. According to the most recent analysis of the American Veterinary Medical Association electronic database, 3.7% of veterinarians in the United States 75 years of age or younger worked in local, state, and federal governmental agencies, with only 3.9% of private clinical veterinarians serving in food animal exclusive capacities.[16] From a practical standpoint, postgraduation most practitioners do not have the time or flexibility to spend taking lengthy classes and workshops that teach them how to be involved in disaster management. Many are hesitant to attend training that may never be used. Because of time restraints, priority for continuing education (CE) is often given to prevalent conditions and diseases. Furthermore, there may also be a lack of funding to support veterinary training and education. Although many of the state and federally sponsored disaster management courses offered are free of charge, funds for travel and monies to hire a relief veterinarian or otherwise earn a wage while training are rarely available.

DISCUSSION AND RECOMMENDATIONS
Readiness for a Foreign Animal Disease

Awareness
Disaster management includes disaster readiness, disaster response, and disaster recovery. Each play an important role in the overall successful mitigation of an animal disaster, but disaster readiness, including awareness and preparedness, is the most important phase that guides response and recovery activities. Disaster readiness begins with an awareness of potential hazards or events to which communities are susceptible. Veterinary practitioners that cover large geographic areas, work in areas that include an international border, or include large numbers of food animals in their practice specifically need to begin preparations for a potential FAD introduction before an actual event. Veterinarians have some familiarity with FADs through their initial veterinary schooling and subsequent accreditation renewals. It is imperative that they remain vigilant and current with US and global incursions, because the global animal health situation is constantly changing.

On a daily basis, practitioners treat a variety of clinical cases and are expected to practice preventive medicine, recognize disease trends, consult on morbidities, and educate producers. The ability to recognize the potential threat of an FAD intrusion most likely rests on a veterinary practitioner doing their normal, everyday calls when "something different" is seen. Repeated CE courses on FAD recognition strengthen the practitioner's ability to recognize the potential "zebra" if one should occur. In the event of an FAD surfacing in the United States, recognizing the potential threat and initiating the proper response will be the major factor in initial disease containment.

The USDA APHIS is the lead agency for incident management in an FAD event. Because many states have differing rules and regulations governing the state agency having the authority to rapidly stop livestock movement, practitioners should make themselves aware of the specific animal health officials and agencies that would need to be contacted if a suspicious disease were encountered.[17] In some states, regulatory livestock boards or agencies may hold the authority to stop movement, so practitioners need to familiarize themselves with the organizational hierarchy of their animal regulatory agencies, and who the contact would be in each agency if suspicion of an FAD introduction occurs. If an agroterrorism or bioterrorism event is suspected, the FBI takes the lead in the investigation.

Veterinary practitioners should also recognize that their skills extend beyond the traditional veterinary medical care that they are used to providing. In addition to animal diseases, practitioners have unique training in such areas as epidemiology, food safety, animal care/welfare, environmental health, and preventive medicine. Furthermore, veterinarians are able to recognize the importance of the human-animal bond and can comprehend social and psychological issues in the event of a disease outbreak. Along with the standard and expected veterinary care, veterinarians can also contribute leadership, organization, and communication skills to the management of an FAD. Not only is it important for veterinarians to be aware of their role in a community disaster, but first responders and emergency managers at the local, state, and federal levels need to be aware of the important contributions veterinarians can make in disaster management. As the saying goes, a disaster is the wrong time to exchange business cards, so practitioners should become active in the community and surrounding areas before an outbreak or other event occurs so that everyone involved in a response is familiar with each other's capabilities and resources.

Preparedness
Preparedness includes the necessary training and exercises to respond to an FAD. States with a veterinary response team or SART should provide practitioners with

the necessary training and instruction to respond to a potential threat. Such programs as the Arizona Livestock Incident Response Team (ALIRT) or the New Mexico Ag/Livestock Incident Response Team (NM-ALIRT) are examples of state-level first responder groups that involve veterinary practitioners and allied industry partners that train and exercise potential FAD intrusions.[18] The objective is to bring people who will be responding together to train together for a more efficient response. Members are invited to training based on their availability and interests. These groups exist to respond to large or suspicious livestock losses that occur within the state, and whose primary function is to gather information, specimens, video and photographic evidence, assess the situation, and make a judgment as to the level of response needed in each particular case. The joint training of these two state-level response groups provides a regional response network. The idea is to assist in a rapid and accurate diagnosis of the causative agent for the livestock loss, but also to initiate a higher-level response if deemed necessary. Such groups as ALIRT and NM-ALIRT provide equipment kits that are a grab-and-go kit with everything needed to perform multiple necropsies and gather multiple specimens and information to assist in the rapid diagnosis process (personal communication, J.C. Wenzel, State Coordinator, NM-ALIRT).

Advanced training in such areas as disease detection and diagnosis, biosecurity, PPE, decontamination, depopulation, and disposal is essential in the successful mitigation of an outbreak. Knowledge of the principles of biosecurity is used in every aspect of a disease response. Veterinary first responders need to understand the principles, proper use, and disposal of PPE so they are protected if a zoonotic component to the disease response is included. Responders need to practice using PPE, so they do not contribute to the spread of disease in the event of a disease response.[19]

A limited but growing number of veterinary schools provide disaster training and education as part of the core curriculum, electives, postgraduate programs, or other organizational activities.[20,21] In North Carolina and Texas, for example, disaster preparedness education has been a required component of the DVM curriculum since 2002 and 2012, respectively.[20,22] The University of Florida's College of Veterinary Medicine is also a lead member of their SART team, maintaining a fully deployable resource of faculty, staff, and student volunteers since 2004. Several colleges of veterinary medicine, such as Mississippi State University and Texas A&M University, are actively involved in their state's Veterinary Medical Reserve Corps and serve as the main deployable veterinary medical resource in the state. However, standard publications or presentations on the topic of disaster response are lacking in veterinary schools, indicating the need for more integrated emergency management training.

Core competencies for human health professions have been recommended[23]; however, similar suggestions for veterinarians and veterinary students have only recently emerged.[22] The Association of American Veterinary Medical Colleges recognizes the importance of education in emergency management and has made recommendations to the standardized veterinary curriculum to reflect this position.[24] In addition, the USDA National Veterinary Accreditation Program now incorporates a module on animal health emergency response that veterinarians can take to become educated in such areas as the Incident Command System (ICS), National Incident Management System, and the roles of various organizations and agencies.[25,26]

Additional training opportunities have become available to veterinarians through online resources and learning modules (**Table 1**), veterinary CE programs, and locally supported exercises. Cross-training with other local, state, and tribal entities who may have funded programs in place is another way to receive training. Many traditional first responder agencies have training budgets that can accommodate additional

Table 1
Training resources for veterinarians

Resource, Description	Online Information
American Veterinary Medical Association Veterinary First Responder Certificate Program	https://www.avma.org/resources-tools/animal-health-and-welfare/disaster-preparedness/avma-veterinary-first-responder-certificate-program
Center for Food Safety and Public Health Just-in-Time training provides animal diseases resources for veterinarians and first responders	https://www.cfsph.iastate.edu/emergency-response/just-in-time-training/
FEMA Independent Study Program training modules, including: • Incident Command: ICS 100, 200, 700 • Animals in Disasters: IS 10a, IS 11a • Livestock in Disasters: 111a	https://training.fema.gov/is/crslist.aspx?lang=en
Michigan State University Veterinarian Training and Preparedness for Foreign Animal Disease on-line course	https://www.canr.msu.edu/courses/veterinarian-training-and-preparedness-for-foreign-animal-disease
National Animal Health Emergency Management System provides detailed planning resources for critical preparedness and response activities that provide veterinary authority for responders, planners, and policy-makers	https://www.aphis.usda.gov/aphis/ourfocus/animalhealth/emergency-management/ct_nahems_em_guidelines
The Secure Food Supply Plans are commodity-specific plans that use science-and risk-based information to facilitate market continuity for specific products, such as meat and milk, in an outbreak • Secure Beef Supply https://www.securebeef.org/ • Secure Milk Supply https://securemilksupply.org/	https://www.cfsph.iastate.edu/secure-food-supply
USDA APHIS Foreign Animal Disease Preparedness and Response Plans (FAD PReP) contain standard operating procedures and provide information on critical activities conducted during an animal health emergency	https://www.aphis.usda.gov/aphis/ourfocus/animalhealth/emergency-management/!ut/p/z1/fYs9D4IwEIZ3foULo7mSGNSRoPEzztClOaFAtRxQqoF_LyFEXfSG9yv3AHdmM24iIYwxEl-OXDCp8rRqopQQwQx98XFC3mFX9SG9yv3AHdmM24iIYwxEl-OXDCp8rRqopQQwQx98XFC3dstfDOu-3GY8F-FTjtlz5joQfHEfzw3wL8PxtN7PT-NojVrWl4ADypyMrOQoR1o VoxVrJCq6tB07usRVE9jMiq5NGODUmVqEUhUdtiXGQpTS4p 6UWJhPlQybosw3ReG1m7TFEqO6jvPH4B0GTgLwI!/

responders or volunteers, and veterinarians can add and enhance their knowledge and skills in animal and public health in an integrated community response.

There are many postgraduation disaster management training opportunities available for veterinarians starting with the basic National Incident Management System and ICS requirements to comply with official emergency management standards. ICS is used by the government under the National Response Framework, where varying agencies involved in a disaster response fall into an organized structure for response.[27] Basic ICS training is necessary to understand the language, organization, and roles of each responder to an incident that is managed under ICS, as would occur in an FAD intrusion. Courses are available online that provide adequate instruction on ICS, and participating in exercises that use ICS are invaluable training opportunities.

Many veterinary state boards now recognize the value of disaster management training and offer CE credits for their completion. CE credits are required for license renewal for veterinarians.[28] Exercises that bring together veterinarians and first responders are becoming increasingly more common and offer opportunities for collaboration between emergency management, public health, and veterinary medicine. However, this type of training is not always easily understood or accomplished; according to one survey, veterinarians wanted self-paced training because of time constraints of daily clinical practice and family obligations, with a focus on what they specifically would do in a response, not just generic preparedness training.[29] In response to the needs of the profession, the American Veterinary Medical Association has developed a Veterinary First Responder Certificate Program to offer core courses in skills needed to effectively and efficiently respond to a disaster.[30]

Continuity of operations

Disaster readiness should occur at personal, business, and community levels. Continuity of operations can include processes necessary to continue critical functions at home, at the clinic/practice, and at veterinary clients' businesses. At minimum, veterinarians should have a disaster plan for themselves and for their families. When volunteering to assist beyond their personal circle, veterinary responders should make sure their own families and animals will be cared for during a disaster so that other first responders and resources are not taxed further by caring for them in their absence. If they have livestock at home, they should be prepared to minimize contact and make provisions to have other family members or neighbors care for their animals, which could include making arrangements for biocontainment, quarantine and isolation, transportation, and food, water, and shelter provisions, as necessary.

Business continuity is the term used to describe planning and preparedness activities to ensure a business's critical functions will continue despite serious incidents, such as a disease outbreak, that might interrupt them.[17] Practitioners should be aware of local resources so that they can continue to provide needed services to their community by having disaster plans in place for their practice and clientele. Policies and procedures should be developed to continue necessary veterinary services in the event of an FAD. Strategies to ensure critical coverage during a disease outbreak may include performing biosecurity risk assessments before every farm call, staggering coverage with associates or between clinics, cleaning and disinfection of all vehicles and equipment between each farm call, and workforce contingency planning in the event of an FAD exposure. In addition to ensuring the availability of veterinary care, locate an area where patients can be securely and safely housed, such as an enclosed livestock arena or isolated paddock. Furthermore, having a communication plan is especially important in an ambulatory situation, where communication is unreliable even on a good day because cellular service is often unstable in rural areas. Furthermore, the mobile nature of ambulatory practice intensifies the need for biosecurity, and veterinarians must be able to communicate with regulatory officials and their own clients in the event of an FAD outbreak.

Practitioners are instrumental in minimizing disruptions to their livestock clients caused by disease outbreaks by helping them prepare farm-specific disaster plans. Several planning resources based on performing on-farm risk assessments and evaluating biosecurity practices have been made available in recent years to livestock producers and veterinarians.[31,32] Chances are, in a large FAD outbreak, livestock commodities, such as meat, milk, and cheese, will need to stay in commerce to avoid a food chain disruption. The Secure Food Supply plans offer templates for practicing biosecurity on livestock operations and serve as a great resource for farm-specific planning for continuity of operations if an event were to occur.[32] The Secure Beef Supply and Secure Milk Supply plans are specific to ensuring cattle products are minimally affected. Practitioners can actively engage clients through the completion of a Secure Food Supply plan while strengthening their veterinarian-client patient relationship. Furthermore, enhanced biosecurity plans may be required when appropriate to allow permitted movement of livestock in the event of a mandated stop-movement order. Readers should reference the previous *Veterinary Clinics of North America: Food Animal Practice* article titled "Foreign Animal Disease Outbreaks" (July 2018) for additional information on business continuity.[17]

In the event of disease where animal movements will be stopped or strictly regulated, planning for feed and water supplies will likely involve the neighboring farms and ranches, and local livestock event facilities. Livestock should be kept current on their vaccinations to protect them if they need to be moved quickly. Permanent animal identification should be used to prevent livestock from being lost or stolen. In feeder-type operations, producers should know how much feed is on hand or available should there be a disruption in the transportation chain.

Response to a Foreign Animal Disease

In the event of an outbreak, the immediate goal is the detection, control, and containment of the FAD, followed by eradication and facilitation of the continuity of business for noninfected animals and animal products.[33] The practitioner has an important role in all of these activities. Practitioners are the first line of defense in the detection, control, and containment of the FAD, being the first to recognize disease sentinels through frontline surveillance. They are expected to educate producers on the disease and biosecurity practices necessary to prevent and control the outbreak and may be asked to work with local extension personnel to ensure factual and timely messaging gets done. Finally, in the event of a large outbreak, they may be employed by the government during the disease response to assist in continued disease control and surveillance activities, such as performing investigations, animal tracebacks, diagnostic testing, decontamination, and depopulation (additional disease investigation and response considerations are discussed elsewhere in this issue).

Practitioners trained in disaster response are better able to provide a quick assessment that may result in an appropriate response, and it is hoped, containment of a potential disease threat. Training, and participating in exercises that use that training, as discussed in the previous section, is the only way to become proficient and confident of the steps involved in the response process. The practitioner who suspects an unusual condition or FAD should err on the side of caution and contact animal health officials to report the occurrence. If an FAD is suspected on a farm or in a livestock facility, the following succession of events is likely to occur (**Fig. 1**):

- The state and federal veterinarians should be among the first notified of a suspicious disease.
- The practitioner will be provided with advice for further action until investigation is completed.
- If warranted by history and clinical signs of the affected animals, a trained FAD diagnostician will be dispatched. They may or may not collect samples for submission.
- Depending on the scope and distribution of the FAD, stop movement orders, animal quarantine, and other business interruptions may occur.

When an FAD is confirmed, the USDA is the lead agency managing the outbreak, with the state having jurisdiction over stop-movement and quarantine authority.[17] The USDA may activate an Incident Management Team to help manage the overall disease response. An Incident Commander is tasked with setting priorities and providing oversight of the response. The role of accredited veterinary practitioners

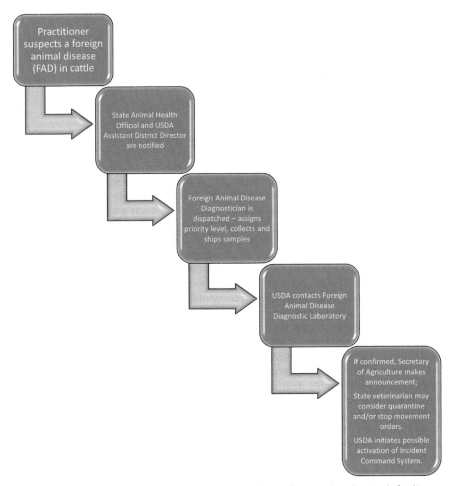

Fig. 1. Succession of events in case FAD is suspected on a farm or in a livestock facility.

depends on the level and extent of their response training, the magnitude and duration of the response, and the availability of response-trained personnel. Understanding the ICS Command structure greatly increases the effectiveness of the practitioner in responding to assigned roles. First responders, including veterinarians, who are dispatched to an incident who have not been ICS trained are a detriment to the process and may be asked to leave the scene. Just-in-Time training is a need-related training that may be used to quickly train responders in the face of an FAD outbreak.

When the disease response is just beginning, practitioners who arrive on-site first may be given more responsibility, then relieved and reassigned when better-trained personnel arrive at the scene. Accredited practitioners that have been involved in training and exercises are given more responsibility in the response organizational chart. Some practitioners who have extensive training may be included in the command structure as subject matter experts, or possibly as an operations section chief or group leader. Once a response is underway, accredited practitioners may be used out in the field carrying out specific objectives of the operational plan, which is the level at which the actual disease response work is carried out. Practitioners and their response teams may be asked to perform a variety of duties, including

- Assessing morbidity
- Treating and caring for the affected animals
- Management and biocontainment of infected premises
- Documentation and surveillance of animals present
- Performing emergency vaccination
- Collecting specimens and necropsying mortalities
- Performing euthanasia and carcass disposal

The practitioner's role generally is to accomplish specific tasks in each operational period, as assigned by the direct supervisor within the ICS structure. It is important to understand that when involved in a response framework, specific tasks are given, and veterinary responders are not to stray from the assigned tasks. Practitioners who volunteer beyond their practice obligations may be asked to sign a code of conduct agreement with the lead response agency that covers such areas as professional conduct, confidentiality, media requests, and photography.[34]

Although biosecurity principles generally should be practiced on a daily basis by practitioners, it is imperative to use enhanced biosecurity practices when an FAD is suspected. Adequate stocks of PPE, in addition to the proper amount and types of disinfectants, should be maintained, properly used, and disposed of after use.[19] Responders may be asked to assist in biosecurity enforcement at a scene. Disease control zones around an infected premises, including infected, buffer, quarantine, and surveillance zones are established.[33,35] Equipment and veterinary supplies taken to a scene by responders need to be labeled because items used on an infected premises may have to be left on-scene to be cleaned and disinfected and retrieved later. Some diseases, such as FMD, require that responders do not leave the premise until proper cleaning and disinfection stations are operational, so veterinary responders need to be prepared to remain on-site.

Practitioners may also be involved in epidemiologic surveillance and investigation. Monitoring human, animal, and traffic movements helps with any trace-backs that may need to be performed. Furthermore, as restrictions are lifted, practitioners may be involved in performing risk assessments, animal inspections, and issuing permits or certificates of veterinary inspection for movement of animals and animal products.

If intentional or criminal introduction of the causative biologic agent is suspected, such as in a bioterrorism event, crime scene preservation techniques need to be used. Instruction and training from law enforcement agencies, such as the FBI, are invaluable to make sure no criminal evidence is destroyed in the initial response process. The FBI has many resources used in training and have been willing to train veterinary first responders in such topics as crime scene preservation, approach to a crime scene, how to preserve evidence, chain of custody of specimens, and resources that the FBI can "bring to the table" in response to an event with possible criminal intent. The contact for such training is the local weapons of mass destruction coordinator. Some states also have an Infragard chapter, which is led by the FBI but is open to the private sector as an outlet for education, information-sharing, networking and technology-sharing regarding threats to areas of critical infrastructure, such as agriculture.

Cooperation and collaboration at all levels is critical to the successful mitigation of a disaster event. Local law enforcement and community leaders rely on practitioners to assist with the implementation of livestock quarantine and stop movement orders. In such cases where other agencies may be helping with movement control or animal handling, the veterinarian may be responsible for on-site or Just-in-Time training of other first responders in the basic principles of not only biosecurity but animal behavior (eg, understanding of flight zones) and animal welfare.

SUMMARY

The threat of FADs is steadily increasing given the ease of international trade and transport, and these diseases have the potential for significant losses to the US cattle industry. Disaster readiness, which includes awareness and preparedness, is the most important phase of disaster management that guides response and recovery activities. Preparing for and responding to the needs of cattle operations in the face of an FAD is resource-intensive and beyond what is provided by most local and state jurisdictions. It is incumbent on livestock veterinarians to remain prepared to respond to FADs through relevant and rigorous training. They should also help their clients develop Continuity of Operations or Emergency Plans that are designed to limit the financial losses and compromised animal welfare that occurs when livestock are exposed or affected with an FAD. Veterinary practitioners should participate in the development of public emergency plans focused on limiting losses in the cattle industry.

CLINICS CARE POINTS

- Awareness of and preparedness for a potential FAD drives an effective and efficient response.
- Training in the proper use of personal protective equipment and disinfectants is imperative to stop the spread of disease.
- Accredited practitioners should be prepared to do a variety of activities, from cleaning and disinfection to education and emergency vaccine and delivery.
- The development of enhanced biosecurity plans helps prevent the introduction of diseases, reduce transmission of disease, and support business continuity in the event of an FAD outbreak.

DISCLOSURE

The authors have nothing to disclose.

REFERENCES

1. USDA National Agriculture Statistics Service. https://downloads.usda.library.cornell.edu/usda-esmis/files/j3860694x/gq67m183k/np194m208/2021_Agricultural_Statistics_Book.pdf. Published 2021. Accessed July 25, 2023.
2. Knight-Jones TJD, Rushton J. The economic impacts of foot and mouth disease: what are they, how big are they and where do they occur? Prev Vet Med 2013;112(3–4):162–73.
3. Carpenter TE, Christiansen LE, Dickey BF, et al. Potential impact of an introduction of foot-and-mouth disease into the California State Fair. J Am Vet Med Assoc 2007;231(8):1231–5.
4. Mort M, Convery I, Baxter J, et al. Animal disease and human trauma: the psychosocial implications of the 2001 UK Foot and Mouth Disease disaster. J Appl Anim Welfare Sci 2008;11(2):133–48.
5. Kester WO, Miller EB. Veterinary aspects of atomic explosion. J Am Vet Med Assoc 1948;325–9.
6. USDA APHIS. National Veterinary Accreditation Program: History of the Program. https://www.aphis.usda.gov/aphis/ourfocus/animalhealth/nvap/ct_history. Accessed October 11, 2016.
7. USDA APHIS. National Veterinary Accreditation Program: Module 19: Animal Health Emergency Response. http://aast.cfsph.iastate.edu/AHER/index.htm.
8. Oladosu G, Rose A, Lee B. Economic impacts of potential foot and mouth disease agroterrorism in the USA: a general equilibrium analysis. J Bioterrorism Biodefense 2013. https://doi.org/10.4172/2157-2526.S12-001.
9. Carriquiry M, Elobeid A, Hayes D. National impacts of a domestic outbreak of foot and mouth disease and African swine fever in the United States. Ames, IA: Working Paper 23-WP 650; 2023. https://www.card.iastate.edu/products/publications/pdf/23wp650.pdf.
10. Evans B. Emergency preparedness: community challenge and obligation. Can Vet J 2002;43:797.
11. American Veterinary Medical Association. Disaster preparedness for veterinarians. 2018. Available at: https://www.avma.org/KB/Resources/Reference/disaster/Pages/default.aspx. [Accessed 4 January 2018].
12. Heath SE, Hooks J, Marshall K, et al. Participation of veterinarians in disaster management. J Am Vet Med Assoc 1997;210(3):325–8.
13. Nolen RS. Wildlife rescue under way as oil gushes into Gulf. J Am Vet Med Assoc 2010;237(2):2.
14. Spain CV, Green RC, Davis L, et al. The national capabilities for animal response in emergencies (NCARE) study: an assessment of US states and counties. J Homel Secur Emerg Manag 2017;14(3):1–14.
15. Guerdan BR. Disaster preparedness and disaster management: the development and piloting of a self-assessment survey to judge the adequacy of community-based physician knowledge. Am J Clin Med 2009;6(3):32–40.
16. American Veterinary Medical Association. US veterinarians. 2022. Available at: https://www.avma.org/resources-tools/reports-statistics/market-research-statistics-us-veterinarians. [Accessed 15 September 2023].
17. Bickett-Weddle DA, Sanderson MW, Parker EJ. Foreign animal disease outbreaks. Vet Clin North Am - Food Anim Pract 2018;34(2):341–54.

18. Extension AC. AZ Livestock Incident Response Team. https://extension.arizona.edu/alirt. Accessed July 23, 2023.
19. Wenzel JGW, Nusbaum KE. Veterinary expertise in biosecurity and biological risk assessment. J Am Vet Med Assoc 2007;230(10):1476–80.
20. Dunning D, Martin P, Tickel JL, et al. Preparedness and disaster response training for veterinary students: literature review and description of the North Carolina State University Credentialed Veterinary Responder Program. J Vet Med Educ 2009;36(3):317–30.
21. Huston CL. Training veterinarians in disaster management using a One Health approach. Alexandria, VA: Annual meeting of the American association of veterinary medical colleges; 2014.
22. Bissett WT, Zoran DL, Clendenin A, et al. How a disaster preparedness rotation helps teach the seven NAVMEC professional competencies: the Texas A&M University experience. J Vet Med Educ 2013;40(4):378–88. https://login.proxy.library.msstate.edu/login?url=http://search.ebscohost.com/login.aspx?direct=true&db=edswsc&AN=000326889400010&site=eds-live.
23. Markenson D, DiMaggio CJ, Redlener IE. Preparing health professions students for terrorism, disaster, and public health emergencies: Core competencies. Acad Med 2005;80(6):517–26. https://login.proxy.library.msstate.edu/login?url=http://search.ebscohost.com/login.aspx?direct=true&db=edsbas&AN=edsbas.ftcolumbiauniv.academiccommons.columbia.edu.ac.155696&site=eds-live.
24. Willis NG, Monroe Fa, Potworowski JA, et al. Envisioning the future of veterinary medical education: the Association of American Veterinary Medical Colleges Foresight Project, Final Report. J Vet Med Educ 2007;34(1):1–41.
25. Torres A, Bowman QP, AVMA-USDA Relations Committee. New directions for the National Veterinary Accreditation Program. J Am Vet Med Assoc 2002;220(10):1470–2.
26. Wenzel JGW, Wright JC. Veterinary accreditation and some new imperatives for national preparedness. J Am Vet Med Assoc 2007;230(9):4.
27. US Department of Homeland Security. National Response Framework. https://www.fema.gov/media-library/assets/documents/32230.
28. Nusbaum KE, Rollin BE, Wohl JS. The veterinary profession's duty of care in response to disasters and food animal emergencies. J Am Vet Med Assoc 2007;231(2):200–2.
29. Hsu CE, Jacobson H, Feldman K, et al. Assessing bioterrorism preparedness and response of rural veterinarians: experiences and training needs. J Vet Med Educ 2008;35(2):262–8.
30. American Veterinary Medical Association. AVMA Veterinary First Responder Certificate Program. https://www.avma.org/resources-tools/animal-health-and-welfare/disaster-preparedness/avma-veterinary-first-responder-certificate-program. Accessed July 23, 2023.
31. Beef Quality Assurance. Daily Biosecurity Plan for Disease Prevention. https://www.bqa.org/Media/BQA/Docs/bqa-daily-biosecurity-plan_12-04-2020-93.pdf. Accessed July 23, 2023.
32. Secure beef supply: biosecurity resources for producers. https://www.securebeef.org/beef-producers/biosecurity/. Accessed July 25, 2023.
33. USDA APHIS VS. FAD PReP National Animal Health Emergency Management System: quarantine and movement control. 2016. Available at: https://www.aphis.usda.gov/animal_health/emergency_management/downloads/nahems_guidelines/nahems_qmc.pdf. [Accessed 25 July 2023].

34. National Alliance of State Animal and Agriculture Emergency Programs. Current best practices in animal emergency management disaster veterinary medical response. 2023. Available at: https://www.thenasaaep.com/nasaaep-best-practice-working-groups. [Accessed 15 September 2023].
35. Wenzel JGW. Awareness-level information for veterinarians on control zones, personal protective equipment, and decontamination. J Am Vet Med Assoc 2007; 231(1):48–51.

The Global Framework for the Progressive Control of Transboundary Animal Diseases - Strengthening Infectious Disease Management and Veterinary Systems Across the Continents

Origins and Testimony

Juan Lubroth, BA, MSc, DVM, PhD, ACVPM*

KEYWORDS

- Rinderpest • Foot-and-mouth disease • Emerging diseases
- Transboundary animal diseases • Foreign animal diseases
- International collaboration • Animal disease management
- Food and Agriculture Organization (FAO)

KEY POINTS

- Tackling the disease at source, Progressive disease management, Risk based interventions, Interregional veterinary networks, International veterinary cooperation.

Transboundary animal diseases are defined by the Food and Agriculture Organization (FAO) of the United Nation's Emergency Prevention System (EMPRES) as those diseases that are of significant economic, trade and/or food security importance for considerable number of countries, which can easily spread to other countries and reach epidemic proportions, and where control/management including exclusion requires cooperation among several countries.[1] The Global Framework for the Progressive Control of Transboundary Animal Diseases (GF-TADs)[2,3] represents a platform of the FAO and World Organisation for Animal Health (WOAH; previously known as the OIE—*Office International des Epizooties*) signed in 2004 to engage regional subregional organizations and national veterinary authorities in developing and monitoring progress in animal disease management efforts and mutual cooperation to address animal health priorities and disease threats.[3] Included in the GF-TADs are aspects

Lubroth One Health Consultancies, Casaprota, Italy
* Corresponding author.
E-mail address: Jlubroth@gmail.com

Vet Clin Food Anim 40 (2024) 233–249
https://doi.org/10.1016/j.cvfa.2024.01.009
0749-0720/24/© 2024 Elsevier Inc. All rights reserved.

related to enhanced surveillance and reporting, the development and institution of the Global Early Warning System (with the World Health Organization [WHO]),[4] capacity building within diagnostic laboratory facilities, emergency preparedness and response, and establishment of regional networks for capacity building, sharing of information, and measuring progress.

BACKGROUND AND HISTORY

At the turn of the millennium, several outbreaks of foot-and-mouth disease (FMD) captured international headlines. Outbreaks in the United Kingdom, France, the Netherlands, Ireland, Republic of Korea, Japan, Argentina, and Uruguay led national authorities to counter the spread of one of the most infectious diseases known to medicine through massive culls, the construction of burial pits and pyres, halting trade across multiple agricultural products, as well as curbing tourism, trade, and travel. The prevailing international practices of countermeasures—considered best practices—came under public and national scrutiny calling into question the draconian methodologies. Even other national veterinary services and private sector interests in countries that were not affected by the FMD outbreaks took notice of the public outcry and reviewed their emergency preparation and contingency plans, including the establishment of regulations where vaccination could be incorporated into FMD outbreak countermeasures (ie, "vaccination-to-live" policies), rather than total elimination of affected and potential susceptible populations.[5]

The author at the time was Head of the Reagents and Vaccines Unit and Manager of the North American FMD Vaccine Bank (and previous Head of the Diagnostic Services Section) at the Plum Island Animal Disease Center, a research and diagnostic laboratory facility of the United States Department of Agriculture's Agricultural Research Service and the Animal and Plant Health Inspection Service, off the coast of New York and Connecticut. In 2001, he was recruited by the Food and Agriculture Organization (FAO) of the United Nations' (UN's) Animal Health Service as Head of Infectious Diseases/Emergency Prevention System (EMPRES), with one of the responsibilities being to develop a special program for the eradication of FMD. Over the next 36 months, working with other specialists at FAO and some of its global and regional Reference Centers, the concept of FMD elimination/eradication expanded to include priority diseases that shared similar characteristics with FMD: those highly transmissible animal diseases that impact food security, people's livelihoods, economic development, and threats to safe trade.

THE COMPLEXITY OF FOOT-AND-MOUTH DISEASE

FMD viruses cause several diseases that are characterized by similar clinical signs and pathologic features in livestock (See Chapter 1). Some strains have broad host ranges, including wildlife, and others more specific host "preferences" or tropisms. One characteristic of the FMD viruses is their genetic, antigenic variability and their geographic footprint, which required that vaccines produced be tested against the prevailing circulating serotypes and strains. Thus, the multiple host range, antigenic variability, high transmission rates in susceptible populations, carrier state in certain species, and geographic endemic presence [since 1900 through 2000] in large swaths of Africa, the Middle East, South America, Asia, and eastern Europe remained of great concern to authorities of countries free from the disease or those commercial interests that wish to trade in livestock and their commodities (milk and other dairy products, leather, embryos, trophies), but were unable to do so because of the presence of FMD. In the international trade arena of agriculture, and in particular livestock, the presence or absence of FMD has been a determinant in the establishment of regulatory structures and in mitigating threats. Arguably, the 'discovery' of bovine spongiform encephalopathy and its epidemiology linked to feed and food production further added complexity to veterinary regulatory precautions and regulatory framework in global trade.

Thus, in the planning and devolution of a global program for FMD control and elimination[6] — and what would become GF-TADs[4] — breaking down the nature of complexity of FMD and its management offered an opportunity to address and develop competencies to improve overall animal disease management.

ORIGINS AND OBJECTIVES

The FAO/EMPRES precepts of Early Warning, Early Reaction, Enabling Research, and Coordination[7(p8)] and WOAH's mandate in the setting of standards for safe animal trade, official animal disease status of countries was the critical element in the establishment of GF-TADs. Both world bodies—representing close to 200 countries—recognized the essence of a regional (ecosystem, cultural, porous borders, opportunities in trade) approach to existing and emergent threats. The GF-TADs parent organizations led the engagement of the regional and sub-regional organizations (**Table 1**) and national authorities of member countries in developing a vision to address the regional animal health disease threats, developing a monitoring structure, and a mechanism for collaboration. Included in the GF-TADs were aspects related to enhanced surveillance and reporting, the development and institution of the Global Early Warning System (with the WHO in the case of priority zoonoses),[4] capacity building within diagnostic laboratory facilities, emergency preparedness and response contingency arrangements, and developing a monitoring of progress matrix.

In February 2003, an early presentation made by the then-Chief of FAO's Animal Health Service, Yves Cheneau, at the WOAH's Middle East Commission meeting outlined the objectives of GF-TADs: (1) improve food security and incomes of developing countries, (2) safeguard the world livestock industry from repeat shocks of infectious disease epidemics, and (3) Promote safe and globalised trade in livestock and animal products. The GF-TADs concept and its strategies at the time remain valid 20 years later: progressive control of the disease at the *source* of infection and the development and strengthening of Veterinary Services through provisions of Guidelines and Standards, Emergency Preparedness, Information Systems, Laboratory Capability, Effective Response, and Prompt Recovery. It was essential that FAO, a technical and development-focused organization of the UN's partner with the WOAH, the global standard setting body in all areas related to animal health and welfare and formed by delegates representing the Chief Veterinary Officers (CVOs) of all countries. In the GF-TADs' strategic updated paper, the framework is described as "...a coordinating mechanism that brings together the public and private sectors, academia, the general public, and regional and international organisations to assist regions, sub-regions and countries in reaching the goal of preventing, promptly detecting and controlling TADs through a worldwide strategy".[8]

The term 'progressive' was an important concept to include in its title as it was aptly recognized that not all necessary components to disease management and eventual control/elimination would be available at once (ie, diagnostic reagents and technical proficiencies, epidemiologic understanding of transmission and animal movements, knowledge or sequencing of circulating pathogenic strains, risk analysis, geospatial and temporal analyses of disease occurrence, vaccine matching, vaccine availability of certified quality, and sufficient human and financial resources).

Table 1
Principal regional organizations proposed to be incorporated into the GF-TADs

	Geographic Scope	Full Name and Specific URL	Membership (2022–23)
Americas			
PAHO	Continental	Pan-American Health Organization www.paho.org	35 (plus 4 Associate Members)
IICA	Continental	Inter-American Institute for Cooperation in Agriculture www.iica.int	34
CAN	Andean countries	Comunidad Andina de Naciones www.comunidadandina.org	4
CARICOM	Caribbean	Caribbean Commission www.caricom.org	19 (plus 5 Associate Members)
OIRSA	Meso-America and Caribbean	Organización Inter-Regional en Salud Agropecuaria www.oirsa.org	9
CAS	Southern Cone/South America	Consejo Agropecuario del Sur www.consejocas.org	6
Asia			
ASEAN	Southeast Asia	Association of Southeastern Asian Nations www.asean.org	10
ECO	Central Asia	Economic Cooperation Organization www.eco.int	10
SAARC	Southern Asia	South Asia Association for Regional Cooperation www.saarc-sec.org	8
Africa			
AU	Continental	African Union https://au.int	55
UMA	North Africa	Union du Maghreb Arabe mwww.maghrebarabe.org	5
COMESA	Eastern and southern Africa	Common Market for Eastern and Southern Africa www.comesa.int	21

EAC	East Africa	East Africa Community www.eac.int	7
ECOWAS	Western Africa	Economic Community of West African States www.ecowas.int	15
SADC	Southern Africa	Southern African Development Community www.sadc.int	16
Europe			
EU	Western Europe	European Union	27
EU-FMD	Europe and parts of Middle East	European Commission for the Control of FMD www.fao.org/eufmd/en	39
Inter-Regional			
REMESA	Mediterranean	Reseau Mediterranéen de Santé Animale www.fao.org/remesanetwork/remesa/en/	15

Middle East – without a unifying regional organization in the Middle East, GF-TADs utilized the existing regional structures of FAO (Regional Office for the Near East, based in Cairo; 18 members) and WAHO's Middle East Regional (based in Beirut; 20 members), with Israel incorporated into the European theater. The Gulf Cooperation Council (6 countries of the Arabian Peninsula) has proposed to establish a GCC Animal Disease Control body (2020).

To this effect, FAO/EMPRES and the European Commission for the Control of FMD (EuFMD), developed the concept of a Progressive Control Pathway for FMD (PCP-FMD), which was subsequently endorsed by WOAH, and whose internal processes would ultimately determine the country's status (freedom with vaccination or freedom without vaccination at national or sub-national level).[9] The PCP-FMD is a risk and evidence-based approach to guide FMD-endemic countries to improve the management of disease risk, reduce its impacts, and curtail viral transmission. As countries advanced through the stepwise approach, FMD risks would be progressively abated and could reach the WOAH status official recognition of freedom from FMD. The PCP-FMD became a core tool of the Global FMD Control Strategy, offered a mechanism to deliver and monitor the GF-TADs platform, and incorporate the evaluation and capacity development tool: WOAH Performance of Veterinary Services Pathway (PVS).[10] Conceptually, a progressive control pathway would be formulated through a series of defined and agreed stages. In general, the following stages showcase the concept of progressive advancement in disease management, elimination, and possible international recognition.

- Stage 0—there is poor understanding of where the disease is and is not present, vaccination may be haphazardly carried out (if at all), and there is no national plan.
- Stage 1—there are efforts to understand the epidemiologic situation in a country and tabulating occurrence (prevalence and incidence) and a national plan has been devised.
- Stage 2—control activities are introduced/strengthened, including vaccination based on risk assessments, an official control program is in place.
- Stage 3—risks and control options are further identified, emergency responses are coordinated and clinical disease has become absent, though targeted or syndromic surveillance is maintained.
- Stage 4—vaccination may be halted and the country provides evidence that the pathogen of concern is no longer circulating at zonal or national level, and depending on WOAH status, could apply to that organization for international recognition of that status (eg, freedom with vaccination/freedom without vaccination).

In the case of FMD, through GF-TADs regional roadmap meetings, a GF-TADs acceptance process was followed, whereby a requirement for (1) the completion of a self-assessment questionnaire ("progressive control pathway [PCP] checklist") by countries is undertaken and collated information would be standardized so comparisons can be made between countries; (2) an FMD-Working Group would review the questionnaires and assessments made as to progress of the required and recommended inputs and outcomes for a given PCP-FMD Stage, and that the FMD plan was consistent with the specific stage in which the country was claiming to be or was wishing to be considered; (3) the country would provide evidence supporting the self-assessment for peer review; and (4) the Regional Advisory Group (composed of 3 CVOs), or their designees, from the region would make the final recommendation of the stage for that particular country. Yearly monitoring of progress could be visually presented at international meetings as maps (ie, WOAH's General Session of the World Assembly of Delegates) with red/yellow/orange for the early stages leading to green, representing inroads to containment of disease at sub-national and national levels and finally freedom.

Though the PCP is conceptually simplistic in its structure, operationalization with the necessary sustained support is more difficult, as other competing priorities are likely in existence, including the turnover of trained professionals, changes and challenges in political leadership, the agreement and compliance by farmers, ranchers, pastoralists, and allied industries, or the compilation of data and information to be provided to peers and the Regional Advisory Group. As the issue at stake is the transmission of highly infectious diseases, it would be hoped that neighboring countries assist each other as having the disease under poor control in one environment could quickly disrupt the status that the country in a higher stage after peer-recognition (or 'official' freedom) had been achieved. Once eliminated, however, surveillance and maintaining risks analysis of potential re-introduction is paramount.

The PCP-FMD concept paved the way for other diseases of importance to GF-TADs (eg, *peste des petits ruminants* [PPR])[11–15] as the process recognized differences in risk of infection between (and within) infected countries and that affected countries were at different levels in managing such risks. Through a PCP approach, each country would be encouraged to develop national risk reduction strategies, not only for the benefit of the country but also its neighbors and trading partners. Regional roadmap meetings (annual or biennial)—especially successful for FMD and PPR—were essential in maintaining momentum, investment at national and local levels, and evaluate progress in disease occurrence and management or guide operators in corrective measures along an agreed regional roadmap.

GLOBAL FRAMEWORK FOR THE PROGRESSIVE CONTROL OF TRANSBOUNDARY ANIMAL DISEASES PLATFORM AND GOVERNANCE

Two global organizations led the effort for GF-TADs which recognized the need for regional inputs—in terms of priority setting and regional leadership (**Tables 2** and **3**). The tabulation of inputs (ie, training exercises, vaccine procurement, laboratory infrastructure, and reagents, etc.) needed to be quantified with selected outputs (vaccinations, timely investigations, sample submissions, definitive diagnostic, and reporting at national and international levels). To this effect, FAO and the WOAH established a Global Steering Committee and parallels within the regions. Five regional steering committees were formed which were similar but not identical in their formats, empowering regional governance views and priority setting and thus ensuring that regional perspectives were heightened over any global prescription (see **Table 3**). The Global Steering Committee included the presidents of the regional GF-TADs structures, regional representatives of the WOAH Commissions, FAO and WOAH leadership with technical and administrative support from the GF-TADs Secretariat hosted by FAO in Rome, Italy (**Fig. 1**). Select regional organization representatives and potential funding partners were also invited—to further dialogue, open engagement, and attract funding to GF-TADs operations. The Regional Secretariats were hosted by WOAH regional structures (Bamako, Beirut, Buenos Aires, Tokyo, and Sofia) and the European Union (Brussels).

The GF-TADs Secretariat was overseen by a GF-TADs Management Committee and composed of the technical and bipartisan leadership from FAO and WOAH with meetings held several times throughout the year. It was during these meetings that not only technical issues were proposed, but also sustained efforts to seek complementary actions, avoid unwarranted competition or duplication, and responding to vis-à-vis in-country support, regional engagement, and planning.

GF-TADs have undergone several internal and external independent evaluations.[16] The GF-TADs Global Strategy 2021 to 2025 incorporates some of the recommendations of these evaluations and a better understanding of global needs and trends (ie, One Health, UN Sustainable Development Goals[a]).[8]

---

[a] Transforming our world: the 2030 Agenda for Sustainable Development, Department of Economic and Social Affairs (un.org).

DISEASE PRIORITIZATION

It terms of prioritization of diseases, at the outset of GF-TADs, the search and elimination of rinderpest was primordial at the global level, even though the Americas and Oceania had had only 1 outbreak each in the 1920's. The last official outbreak was reported in 2001 (Meeru National Park, Kenya), but it was important that all cases of stomatitis-enteritis (ie, syndromic surveillance) were reported, investigated and rinderpest virus excluded as to the cause. Through the official OIE pathway, FAO's Global Rinderpest Eradication Programme and partners (notably the African Union Inter-African Bureau for Animal Resources [AU-IBAR] in the vast African realm) and many bilateral funding partners assisted countries and regions/ecosystems halt decades of vaccination projects and programs, undertake serologic surveys in non-vaccinated animals to determine viral activity amongst susceptible populations, and investigate the zones where the previous dozen or so outbreaks had been reported. After 10 years of repeated serologic surveys in young non-vaccinated bovids (and wild artiodactyls) in targeted areas where the virus had historically occurred in previous decades and the recognition of countries where the disease was never reported, Global Declaration of Freedom from Rinderpest was made at the 70th General Session of the OIE (Paris, May 2011) and by the UN at FAO's 37th Conference (Rome, June 2011).[17] The other pressing global priority for GF-TADs was FMD, affecting or threatening all continents with varying impacts and risks, and all 5 GF-TADs 'regions' included this disease (see **Table 2**).

With the eradication of rinderpest, 1 question frequently asked was "what is next?" And often the answer may have been PPR[b] and FMD, but in developing the strategies for PPR or FMD, it was essential that it would not be seen as disease hopping and thereby neglect other diseases that were local or regional priorities, and that through adjusted inputs, one could also improve overall animal health for the target species (eg, in the case of PPR, interventions to address brucellosis [*Br melitensis*], sheep pox, goat pox, Rift Valley fever, FMD, contagious caprine pleuropneumonia, improved housing and husbandry, flock/animal identification schemes, etc.) could be made at considerable financial and operational savings.[11]

REGIONAL ANIMAL HEALTH CENTERS

In the design of GF-TADs to improve regional outreach, technical and specific project administrative inputs from FAO and WOAH specialists was sought, and Regional Animal Health Centers (RAHC) were established—ideally to be embedded within select regional organizations—to link global projects with tailored regional technical needs and attract local potential funding partners, though in some instances these hubs were hosted by existing FAO or WOAH structures. With the expanding occurrence of H5N1, highly pathogenic avian influenza (H5N1 HPAI), and multilateral funding streams, RAHCs were quickly established in Bangkok, Bamako, Gaborone, and Nairobi between 2004 and 2005, followed by Panama City in 2007 and subsequently in Kathmandu 2008. Of salient importance were veterinary epidemiologists, laboratory specialists, project managers, and communication officers and, depending on available funding (projects), additional specialists could be employed. However, RAHC sustainability was contingent on funding from the regional structures and interested external parties (donors) and in the case of Panama City, Gaborone, and Kathmandu,

---

[b] Petits ruminants, French for small ruminants, in some societies and cultures considered the 'poor people's cattle.'

the RAHCs were short-lived. Nevertheless, the establishment of regional laboratory networks and improvement of laboratory competencies, capacity building exercises in disease search and surveillance, and sharing of information at the regional GF-TADs meetings proved to make important inroads in strengthening national veterinary systems, and in the specific case of avian influenza viruses (some with zoonotic potential) and FMD virus characterization of isolates, allow for better formulation of vaccines (including those for human use through the WHO-OFFLU[c] meetings[18]) and better understanding of viral circulation.

TACKLING THE DISEASE (THREAT) AT SOURCE

Of great importance for GF-TADs was capacity building of the professionals (regulatory, laboratory diagnosticians, clinicians, and even leadership) in management, surveillance activities and reporting, and triggers for improved preparedness. For this the concept of "tackling the disease [or threat[d]] at source" became motto; indicating the importance of risk assessment, syndromic surveillance, early detection, and rapid response—before the infection were to spread across borders and continents, or species barriers.

Understanding threats meant appreciating changing trade patterns and agricultural commodities, climate fluctuations that could affect pathogen-transmitting vectors (eg, bluetongue, Rift Valley fever, lumpy skin disease, Jembrana disease, tick-borne fever/Ehrlichiosis, Cowdriosis/Heartwater, or bovine ephemeral fever), geopolitical instabilities with subsequent refugee migrations, environmental encroachment by extractive industries, or vast public works – could and would provide opportunities to intervene early and institute disease prevention measures. The notion of 'tackling the disease at source' could be interpreted from an ecosystem/geographic point of view as well as from the detection of a disease in a certain host and intervene early before a spillover event could ensue (eg, a zoonotic agent).

AN EARLY WARNING SYSTEM

Though official reporting and notification schemes of disease occurrence at the WOAH and WHO (through the International Health Regulations) have existed prior to advent of GF-TADs, these have certain specificities that are pathogen explicit, whereas the intent in developing a robust Global Early Warning System (GLEWS) for transboundary animal diseases and major zoonoses was to go beyond tabulation of specific pathogens and provide a degree of analysis in the 'warning' as mentioned earlier, that is: drivers to disease emergence or spread. In the GLEWS platform, the 3 international organizations would engage country authorities or key informants for ground-truth investigations and follow-up combined with assisting in sample collection and diagnostic analyses with the support of reference laboratories and other collaborating centers or the provision of information that would alert authorities as to potential instabilities that *may* lead to infection and disease outbreaks (ie, excessive rainfall and likelihood of arthropod-borne disease epidemics, changing trading patterns, or deforestation and other landscape changes). The analysis of changing patterns, climate fluctuations, disruptive public works or those of extractive industries, environmental fragmentation, access to goods and services, is critical to forecast, predict and prevent.

---

[c] OFFLU – WOAH-FAO global network of expertise on animal influenza.

[d] Rather than disease, certain 'threats'—such as antimicrobial resistant pathogens or residues or contaminants could be conceptually included—and their management improved through risk assessments, detection, and appropriate action at source.

Table 2
GF-TADs priority diseases (2004)

Disease	Taxonomic Causative Agent (Species, Genus, Family)
Foot-and-Mouth Disease	Aphthovirus; Picornaviridae
Rinderpest	Morbillivirus; Paramyxoviridae
Peste des Petits Ruminants	Morbillivirus; Paramyxoviridae
Contagious Bovine Pleuropneumonia	*Mycoplasma mycoides* subsp. *mycoides*
Rift Valley Fever	Phlebovirus; Bunyaviridae
Sheep pox/Goat pox	Capripox; Poxviridae
Highly Pathogenic Avian Influenza	Influenza virus; Orthomyxoviridae
African Swine Fever	Asfirvirus; Asfaviridae
Classical Swine Fever	Pestivirus; Flaviviridae
Brucellosis	*Brucella melitensis*
Rabies	Lyssavirus; Rhabdoviridae
Anthrax	*Bacillus anthracis*
Q fever	*Coxiella burnetii*
Bovine Spongiform Encephalopathy	prion
Tularemia	*Francisella tularensis*
Japanese Equine Encephalomyelitis	Flavivirus; Flaviviridae
Venezuelan Equine Encephalomyelitis	Alphavirus; Togaviridae
West Nile Virus	Flavivirus; Flaviviridae
Old World Screwworm	*Chrysomya bezziana*
New World Screwworm	*Cochliomyia hominivorax*
Nipah virus	Henipavirus; Paramyxoviridae
Crimean Congo Hemorrhagic Fever	Orthonairovirus; Nairoviridae
Ebola Virus	Ebolavirus; Filoviridae
Marburg Hemorrhagic Fever	Marburgvirus; Filoviridae
Foodborne diseases	

Of the 25 specific priority animal diseases list of common interest included in the original GF-TADs agreement between FAO and WOAH, 13 infect bovids.

Conceptually, when a disease or pathogen is thought to be eliminated or eradicated, it is essential that syndromic surveillance remains, and the specific pathogen be excluded using laboratory confirmation. The idea that 'the last suspicious case was yesterday, and the next suspected outbreak will be tomorrow' ensures that veterinary professionals and new graduates do not exclude potential recrudescence.

SOLIDARITY

In addressing disease dynamics and continuous threats, a key aspect for FAO, WOAH, and regional groups was the concept of solidarity. Safeguarding national economies and assuring people's livelihoods would benefit all. As such, it would behoove the 'wealthier' countries to advance efforts in improving veterinary service's capabilities around the globe to improve regulatory frameworks, transparency in disease occurrence and management, invest in technology transfer efforts, stimulate collaboration, and ensure safer trade.

The overall strategic insights in the GF-TADs platform were, and are, to augment regional cooperation and shared understanding of common threats (review of

Table 3
Disease priorities by region (see www.gf-tads.org)

Geographic Scope		Primary and Secondary Priority Levels (2004 Initial Priorities with 2022 Updates)
Americas		Foot-and-Mouth Disease, Rabies, Avian Influenza, Bovine Spongiform Encephalopathy, African Swine Fever. Secondary Level: New World Screwworm, Classical Swine Fever.
Africa		Rinderpest (Proof of Freedom), Foot-And-Mouth Disease, African Swine Fever. Secondary Level: Contagious Bovine Pleuropneumonia and Rift Valley Fever
Asia and Pacific	Southeast Asia	Rinderpest (proof of freedom), Foot-and-Mouth Disease, African swine fever, Classical Swine fever, Porcine Respiratory Reproductive Syndrome, Porcine Epidemic Diarrhea, Highly Pathogenic Avian Influenza, and Rabies
	South Asia	Rinderpest (proof of freedom), Foot-and-Mouth Disease, Avian Influenza, Peste des Petits Ruminants, and Rabies
	Pacific	Preventive activities
	East Asia	Rinderpest (proof of freedom), Foot-and-Mouth Disease, African Swine fever, Classical Swine fever, Porcine Respiratory Reproductive Syndrome, Porcine Epidemic Diarrhea, Highly Pathogenic Avian Influenza, and Rabies
Europe		Lumpy Skin Disease, Classical swine fever, African swine fever, Second level of priority: Foot-and-Mouth Disease, Avian Influenza, Brucellosis, and Peste des Petits Ruminants
Middle East		Rinderpest (proof of freedom), Foot-and-Mouth Disease, and Peste des Petits Ruminants. Secondary level: Rift Valley fever, Brucellosis, and Rabies
Global		African Swine Fever, Foot-and-Mouth Disease, Peste des Petits Ruminants, Highly Pathogenic Avian Influenza, and the Rinderpest Post-Eradication Programme

It is to note that priorities have shifted during the initial GF-TADs engagement of 2004 for the countries and their regions, due to eradication (rinderpest and recognition of freedom), effective controls in the previous 20 y (classical swine fever or bovine spongiform encephalopathy) or new recrudescence, new incursions and spread (HPAI and African Swine Fever). Rabies is in reference to dog-mediated virus transmission.

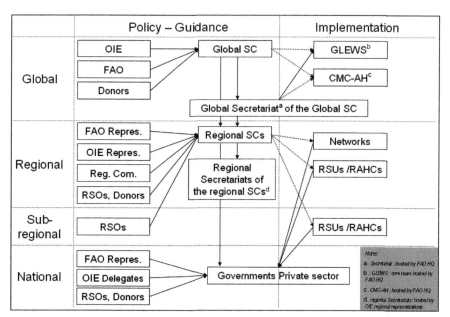

Fig. 1. Governance of GF-TADs as presented during the 5th Global Steering Committee in October 2012, Paris. The GF-TADs Global Secretariat (hosted by FAO, Rome). CMC-AH, Crisis Management Centre-Animal Health (in 2018, the name was changed to Emergency Management Centre-Animal Health); GLEWS, Global Early Warning System (with World Health Organization); RSO, Regional Specialized Organizations; RSU/RAHC, Regional Support Units/Regional Animal Health Centers. WOAH served as the regional Secretariats.

production systems, trade highways, and the joined ecosystems where the select pathogen 'resides') and tackling the disease at source. In having the international and regional organization umbrella, geopolitical feuds—recent, decades, or centenary-old—could be overcome, being that dealing with the common threat improves food security, community livelihoods, safer trade, and national wealth. Under these circumstances and the speed of transcontinental trade of agricultural products occur, including cattle movement, a disease threat anywhere could be in the immediate neighborhood within days, if not hours. Hence, international solidarity and increased financial support are warranted to address action when the problem is localized.

FUNDING DISEASE CONTROL AND ELIMINATION

During the waning years of the rinderpest campaigns in the late 1990's, and as countries and communities had not experienced the devastation of the disease for years, little funding could be attracted to undertake the necessary surveillance to achieve global eradication (ie, the 'last mile'). Through regional engagement (especially that of the AU-IBAR and financial and technical support from the European Commission), the halting of decades-long vaccination campaigns, undertaking the necessary serologic surveys in—presumably non-vaccinated—younger stock and wildlife samples, and rapid reporting of stomatitis-enteritis syndromes could take place.

One of the great stimuli for funding and advancing the GF-TADs platform and its regional approaches was not FMD as the global threat it is, but H5N1 HPAI—with its origins in southern China (1996), rapid spread throughout southeast Asia (2004), followed by Europe, Middle East, and Africa (2006). In addressing the H5N1 avian influenza virus, and because of its zoonotic nature, significant funds were made available to improve medical care, equipment, and veterinary infrastructures and professional competences, as well as improvement in market hygiene, slaughterhouse, transport regulations, or greater cooperation with wildlife specialists. The funds, while earmarked to a certain extent to address HPAI, would nevertheless be valuable to address other emerging or endemic diseases of concern, improve laboratory infrastructure, and provide epidemiologic tools.

As progress is made in pathogen/disease elimination, it would behoove regulatory animal health and those engaged in similar public health disease elimination efforts to identify microbiological and biotechnological research facilities, pharmaceutical interests, faculties of veterinary science, diagnostic clinics and pathology laboratories, and, arguably, defense institutes, in gathering data of historical records of where the pathogen of interest (ie, FMD, rinderpest, PPR, contagious bovine pleuropneumonia [CBPP] was studied or preserved). This effort would be most valuable to ensure the pathogens and derived strains, or their infectious clones, carriers, and pathologic tissues are properly sequestered or destroyed. In the specific case of rinderpest, the effort by FAO and WOAH commenced very late (2009–2010) and precise documentation and historical archives unavailable or lost in the preceding decades when the disease had already been eliminated in some countries and regions. Still, through the concerted efforts of the international and regional organizations through the dissemination of questionnaires to government ministries and faculties of veterinary medicine/research facilities, combined sustained efforts in communication of the importance of proper disposal (destruction) of rinderpest virus or potential rinderpest virus-containing material provided a degree of confidence that not only rinderpest was eradicated from the wild, but also that it would be destroyed or at least contained in approved FAO/WOAH facilities and monitored.[19]

Limited by internal resources of funding, FAO and WOAH sought to attract funding from potential partners to set up a strong GF-TADs mechanism at the global and regional levels. A sustainable source of funding for a GF-TADs Secretariat (administrative personnel, operational resources) and elements in the original concept paper (ie, GLEWS platform, rapid response managers and teams, emergency funds for vaccine procurement and field supplies or equipment, rapid international transport of diagnostic samples to reference laboratories for confirmation or further analysis, regional consultations and meetings) would amount to USD 10 million per annum[3] and its success would save billions of dollars by alerting to a likely threat and responding strategically and timely. Funding to stimulate international cooperation and collaboration remained scarce, as it was apparent that countries, donors, or investors were not as interested in funding the international organizations themselves, but rather preferred to attach their contributions to actual field projects on the ground where inputs, outputs, and outcomes would be more visible. Though understandable from that point of view, it would be incumbent to recognize that coordination and management, including independent and internal evaluations and ensuring complementarity of the diverse project portfolio, at the institutional level would require support the GF-TADs Secretariat with oversights from its Management Committee and guidance from the Global Steering and Regional Committees.

GLOBAL FRAMEWORK FOR THE PROGRESSIVE CONTROL OF TRANSBOUNDARY ANIMAL DISEASES SPINOFFS

Through a strong partnership between FAO and WOAH—and GF-TADs as a platform to address infectious diseases—numerous publications and initiatives were possible.

Some of these include the Global Early Warning System, specific disease consultations, and advice to stakeholders.[e] Others spinoffs include aspects of good practices in livestock health, the Global Rinderpest Action Plan,[19] progressive management pathways for aquaculture biosecurity,[20] terrestrial animal biosecurity,[21] and antimicrobial resistance.[22,23]

In addition, the regional needs to face common threats have led to the creation of regional bodies, much in line with the GF-TADs percepts of collaboration and cooperation, such as REMESA[f] (an animal health network on both sides of the Mediterranean) and the proposed Gulf Cooperation Council's Animal Disease Control Body.[g]

CRITIQUE

The development of a regional cooperation platform to address priority issues, build dialogue and trust between neighbors, is far from new. In the case of animal diseases of an infectious nature, the successes of GF-TADs were—and remain—specific and focused, whereby discussions and recommendations can be converted to action rather than the all-too-often platitudes seen at such international gatherings. However, agreed disease priorities did not include concerns related to transboundary diseases of an aquaculture nature and the present and mounting case regarding antimicrobial resistance (also a multi-host, trade-related and fast spreading, public and food safety issue), which also require a proficient veterinary system to address. It could be argued that a specific strategy and platform be formulated to specifically address these and modeled after GF-TADs.

A second possible critique is the absence of the private sector in the advent and overall governance structure of GF-TADs. However, the private sector represents a vast array of players—family farms to large multinational commercial interests, from pharmaceutical companies to transport associations—thereby diluting the regulatory and legislative framework (a national responsibility) and the required epidemiologic prowess required for progressive control of a priority disease. Though acknowledged, on a myriad of occasions the operators of GF-TADs with their links to FAO and WOAH professionals engaged the private sector for their insight and participation at key sessions in meetings with the condition that their commercial interests or promotion of their enterprise be curtailed. Admittedly, in certain instances, it was a delicate task as preferential treatments to commercial enterprises could be seen as inappropriate.

In line with the above, the GF-TADs concept focused on government veterinary services[h], which in the author's view connotates the official regulatory arm of the veterinary profession and arguably should have used a more comprehensive term referring to veterinary *systems*. This nuance was sought to be important as it expands the regulatory arm with the educational environment, veterinary clinicians and practitioners, hospitals, animal production, and other animal health intervention efforts.

Though technical discussions and strategies may have been largely focused on specific etiologic agents (rinderpest, FMD, PPR, LSD, CBPP and others), to ensure

[e] GF-TADs publications https://www.gf-tads.org/resources/en/.

[f] REMESA - Réseau Méditerranéen de Santé Animale (https://www.fao.org/remesanetwork/remesa/accueil/fr/).

[g] An integrated approach to controlling animal disease outbreaks in the GCC (https://www.strategyand.pwc.com/m1/en/reports/2021/an-integrated-approach-to-controlling-animal-disease-outbreaks-in-the-gcc.html).

[h] In WOAH's glossary, veterinary services is "… combination of governmental and non-governmental individuals and organisations that perform activities to implement the standards of the Terrestrial Code."

that other national or local significant disease problems were addressed and avoid dismissing other diseases of concern, the strategies of GF-TADs would incorporate these and work with tailor-made proposals and options, and include the importance of strengthening veterinary services and systems (ie, WOAH's PVS tool and pathway).[10]

SUMMARY

GF-TADs is a global multilateral, regional initiative and platform to address high impact animal diseases, including salient zoonoses, and led by the global leadership in animal health (FAO of the UN and WOAH) with support from a vast array of reference centers and specialized diagnostic laboratories, other UN bodies, and governed by animal health authorities at country and regional levels. These partnerships have not only led the way to develop progressive control pathways for diseases of global or regional concern, but also an array of platforms and structures (early warning notification, trends analysis, emergency preparedness, and management). In addition, the GF-TADs framework has been instrumental in hosting and labeling global and regional meetings to address specific animal health issues and instruments for disease containment and elimination. While international and government actions to address endemic animal diseases are severely underfunded in comparison to the potential explosive nature of epizootic and transboundary animal diseases, the GF-TADs platform in its initiatives and developed tools help in strengthening veterinary disciplines and regulatory frameworks in the field and in the laboratory to address shortfalls. It has been almost 20 years since GF-TADs was launched with numerous accomplishments, especially cross-border cooperation, international dialogue, and stepwise approaches to improvement (disease status or professional knowledge and competencies). Some important setbacks in disease transcontinental spread have surfaced, notably as African swine fever has shown (2007–2022),[24] but had early appeals for funding been heeded in 2007 the current panorama would likely have been different. Tackling the disease or threat at source is based on early warning, early reporting, and rapid response, and rapid access to needed resources. However, GF-TADs is solely a platform and its success remains with the commitment of countries—government, private sector, producers, and allied industries.

ACKNOWLEDGMENTS

Dozens of people merit appreciation on advancing the GF-TADs across all continents, but in the initial years, special weight and acknowledgments are recognized: Vincent Martin, Andrea Ellis, Julio Pinto, and Karim Ben Jebara (GLEWS); Peter Roeder (Rinderpest); Samia Metwally (post-Rinderpest), Giancarlo Ferrari and Keith Sumption (Progressive Control Pathways); Ian Douglas, Ed Arza, and Lee Myers (preparedness and emergency response); Daniel Chaisemartin and Joseph Domenech (Governance); and, Samuel Jutzi, Bernard Vallat and Monique Eloit (executive support).

DISCLOSURE

The author declares that he has no relevant or material financial interests that relate to the work or prespectives described in this paper. The opinion and views are his alone and should not be considered authoratative FAO views.

REFERENCES

1. Cheneau Y, Roeder PL, Obi TU, et al. Disease prevention and preparedness: the Food and Agriculture Organization Emergency Prevention System. Rev sci tech Off int Epiz 1999;18(1):122–34.
2. FAO. EMPRES Transboundary animal diseases Bulletin 2003; 23. Available at: https://www.fao.org/3/y4809e/y4809e.pdf. [Accessed 16 August 2023].
3. FAO, OIE. Global Framework for the Progressive Control of Transboundary Animal Diseases. 2004. Available at: https://www.fao.org/3/ak136e/ak136e.pdf. [Accessed 15 August 2023].
4. FAO, OIE, WHO. The Global Early Warning and Response System for Major Animal Diseases, including Zoonoses (GLEWS). 2006. Available at: https://www.woah.org/app/uploads/2021/03/glews-tripartite-finalversion010206.pdf. [Accessed 15 August 2023].
5. Orsel K, Bouma A. The effect of foot-and-mouth disease (FMD) vaccination on virus transmission and the significance for the field. Can Vet J 2009;50(10):1059–63.
6. OIE, FAO. The Global Foot and Mouth Disease Control Strategy: Strengthening Animal Health Systems Through Improved Control of Major Diseases. 2012. Available at: www.fao.org/3/an390e/an390e.pdf. [Accessed 15 August 2023].
7. FAO. EMPRES Transboundary animal diseases Bulletin 2002; 21. Available at: https://www.fao.org/3/y3931e/y3931e.pdf. [Accessed 16 August 2023].
8. FAO, WAOH. GF-TADs Strategy for 2021–2025 Enhancing control of transboundary animal diseases for global health. 2022. Available at: https://www.fao.org/3/cb6800en/cb6800en.pdf. [Accessed 15 September 2023].
9. FAO, OIE, EUFMD. The Progressive Control Pathway for Foot and Mouth Disease control (PCP-FMD) - Principles, Stage Descriptions and standards, Second edition. 2018. https://www.fao.org/3/CA1331EN/ca1331en.pdf. [Accessed 15 August 2023].
10. OIE. OIE Tool for the evaluation of performance of veterinary services. 7th edition. Paris: OIE; 2019.
11. OIE, FAO. Global Strategy for the Control and Eradication of PPR. 2015. Available at: www.fao.org/3/I4460E/i4460e.pdf. [Accessed 12 September 2023].
12. El Idrissi A. FAO works to curb the burden of brucellosis in endemic countries Case studies from Eurasia and the Near East, *FAO/EMPRES/Focus on*8. Rome: FAO; 2014.
13. FAO. Developing a stepwise approach for rabies prevention and control. Proceedings of the FAO/GARC Workshop, 2012, Rome, Italy. FAO animal production and health Proceedings, No. 18. Rome, Italy, 2013.
14. WHO, FAO, WOAH. United against Rabies collaboration First annual progress report: global strategic plan to End human Deaths from dog-mediated Rabies by 2030. Rome: WHO, Geneva/FAO; 2019.
15. Diall O, Cecchi G, Wanda G, et al. Developing a Progressive Control Pathway for the control and elimination of African Animal Trypanosomosis. Trends Parasitol 2017;33(7):499–509.
16. FAO and OIE. Evaluation of the global framework for the control of transboundary animal diseases (GF-TADs). FAO, Rome. (www.fao.org/evaluation). Licence: CC BY-NC-SA 3.0 IGO. 2018 www.fao.org/3/CA1959EN/ca1959en.pdf. Accessed August 24, 2023.
17. Taylor WE, Gibbs EPJ, Bandyopadhyay SK, et al. Rinderpest and its eradication. 2022. OIE/Paris and FAO/Rome https://doi.org/10.20506/9789295115606.

18. Edwards S. OFFLU Network on Avian Influenza. Emerg Infect Dis 2006;12(8): 1287–8.
19. Myers L, Metwally S, Marrana M, et al. Global rinderpest action plan post eradication. Paris: FAO, Rome/OIE; 2018. Available at: https://www.fao.org/3/CA1965EN/ca1965en.pdf. [Accessed 11 September 2013].
20. FAO. Report of the Progressive Management Pathway for Improving Aquaculture Biosecurity (PMP/AB): First Technical Working Group Meeting, Rome, 20–22 March 2019. FAO Fisheries and Aquaculture Report No. 1322. ISSN 2070-6987 Rome, Available at: https://doi.org/10.4060/cb0582en. (Accessed 11 September 2023), 2020.
21. FAO. Progressive. Management Pathway for Terrestrial Animal Biosecurity (FAO-PMP-TAB). Rome: FAO; 2023. Available at: https://www.fao.org/3/cc5771en/cc5771en.pdf.
22. FAO. 2021. The FAO action plan on antimicrobial resistance 2021–2025: Supporting innovation and resilience in food and agriculture sectors. Rome, Italy. https://doi.org/10.4060/cb5545en.
23. FAO. Progressive Management Pathway for Antimicrobial Resistance (FAO-PMP-AMR), Available at: https://www.fao.org/antimicrobial-resistance/resources/tools/fao-pmp-amr/en/ (Accessed 15 August 2023).
24. OIE. African swine fever (ASF) report N°47: 2016 – 2020, World Animal Health Information Department, 2020. 2020. Available at: https://www.woah.org/app/uploads/2022/01/asf-situation-report-18062020.pdf. [Accessed 14 September 2023].

Vesicular Stomatitis Virus

Angela M. Pelzel-McCluskey, DVM, MS

KEYWORDS

- Vesicular stomatitis • Livestock disease • Equine • Cattle
- Vector-borne disease outbreak

KEY POINTS

- Vesicular stomatitis (VS) is a disease reportable to state and federal animal health officials in the United States. Veterinarians suspecting VS in a clinical animal should contact either the State Veterinarian or the federal Area Veterinarian in Charge for the state in which the animal is located.
- Diagnostic confirmation of vesicular stomatitis virus (VSV) infection at an approved laboratory is required for the first equine case in a county and in all suspected cases in ruminants and swine.
- Isolation of lesioned animals and implementation of aggressive vector control measures are imperative to reduce the spread of VSV during an outbreak.
- VSV is a zoonotic pathogen, which can be transmitted to humans through direct contact with lesioned animals. Personal protective equipment and good biosecurity practices should be used by veterinarians and animal handlers when handling livestock with active VS lesions.

INTRODUCTION

Vesicular stomatitis (VS) is a viral, vector-borne disease of livestock caused by *Vesiculoviruses*, vesicular stomatitis New Jersey virus (VSNJV) or vesicular stomatitis Indiana virus (VSIV), referred to collectively as vesicular stomatitis viruses (VSVs). The disease is confined to the Americas where it occurs annually in endemic cycles in Mexico, Central America, and northern regions of South America and only in sporadic epizootic outbreaks every 2 to 10 years in the United States.[1] Equids, such as horses, mules, and donkeys, are the most commonly affected species in US outbreaks, followed by cattle and camelids, such as llamas and alpacas[2]; however, the disease can also occur in other ruminants and swine. Clinical signs of the disease in affected species are produced by the development of vesicular (blister-like) lesions that occur on the muzzle, nostrils, lips, oral mucosa, tongue, teats, udder, sheath, ventral abdomen, ears, and/or coronary bands.[3] Lesions in the mouth and on the tongue usually cause hypersalivation and anorexia, whereas coronary band lesions often produce

United States Department of Agriculture, Animal and Plant Health Inspection Service, Veterinary Services, 2150 Centre Avenue, Building B, Fort Collins, CO 80526, USA
E-mail address: Angela.M.Pelzel-McCluskey@usda.gov

lameness. The disease is self-limiting, and the lesions in most affected livestock heal within a couple of weeks without veterinary intervention; however, some older animals or those with underlying health conditions may require supportive care, especially in cases in which the animals cease to eat or drink because of severe oral lesions.[3] The disease is also zoonotic, transmitted to humans through direct contact with infectious lesions in livestock, and typically causes fever, headache, fatigue, and myalgia lasting 3 to 5 days.[3] The appearance of VSV-caused lesions in ruminants and swine is clinically indistinguishable from lesions of foot and mouth disease (FMD), one of the most economically devastating viral diseases of livestock[1]; therefore, immediate reporting to state and federal animal health officials of VSV-like lesions is required in the United States to first rule out FMD infection using appropriate diagnostic assays. Other differential diagnoses in cattle include bluetongue, epizootic hemorrhagic disease, and bovine papular stomatitis.

Transmission of VSV to livestock occurs mainly through biting insects[4]; however, spread can also occur through direct contact with virus-containing fluids from infectious lesions and saliva or through indirect contact with contaminated fomites, such as shared water, feed, feeders, lick tubs, tack, or veterinary supplies, such as oral drenching equipment or dental floats.[5,6] Suspected vectors of VSV include black flies (Simuliidae), sand flies (Psychodidae), and *Culicoides* biting midges (Ceratopogonidae), as species from all 3 of these families have been found naturally infected with VSV in the wild.[7–9] However, other biting insects have been experimentally infected with VSV and may also be involved in transmission. Proximity of affected livestock premises to water has been indicated as a significant risk factor, which is likely reflective of nearness to prime habitat for competent vectors.[10] Black flies hatching from moving waterways and *Culicoides* spp hatching from muddy areas around standing water move directly to nearby livestock to feed thus initiating VSV-transmission in the area if those vector populations are carrying the virus.

Genetic analyses of VSVs from US outbreaks have indicated that they arise from viruses circulating in Mexico.[11–13] Both VSV serotypes and multiple lineages are found circulating in southern and south-central Mexico annually.[1,13,14] It is hypothesized that specific climatic and environmental factors, such as precipitation, temperature, stream flow rates, and vegetative biomass, occur in certain years, which favor the expansion of VSV-carrying vectors northward from these endemic regions.[15] In those years, VS cases are seen in states in northern Mexico just a few months prior to outbreaks being recognized in Texas, New Mexico, and/or Arizona in the United States. These years have been termed incursion years for US outbreaks and the dominant climatological and ecological variables supporting this movement have been modeled and reported.[15] After an incursion year, the virus may overwinter and resurge to cause cases the following year, termed an expansion year, with slightly different climatological and ecological conditions identified as supporting this resurgence.[15] If no VS outbreak is identified in the year following an incursion year, then it is hypothesized that the environmental variables supporting the vectors for an expansion year may not have been present, and therefore continued transmission did not occur. Research is ongoing to further evaluate and understand how climate and ecology affect insect vector populations and the potential for VSV transmission in a given year.

VS outbreaks in the United States cause significant trade disruptions and economic impacts mainly through cessation of international and interstate movement of livestock but also through reduced participation in or cancellation of livestock shows and events[16] and short-term production losses, especially in affected dairy cattle. The seasonality of disease occurrence also has an impact. VS outbreaks occur during the height of vector activity, usually late spring through early fall, which is also the time of year where a high volume of equine shows/events and county fairs are scheduled to occur. Additionally, the large numbers of cattle in the western United States that move through livestock markets and sales in the fall can be held up by VS outbreaks and associated quarantines. States without VS cases issue specific movement restrictions on susceptible livestock species from VS-affected states, which may either bar movement from affected counties altogether or require a certificate of veterinary inspection within just a few days of movement that includes statements by the veterinarian attesting to examination of the animal and the absence of VS lesions. International export of livestock from VS-affected states is halted until at least 30 days after the last quarantine release in the state or longer depending on the requirements of the receiving country. International export of livestock from nonaffected US states is usually able to proceed; however testing for VSV may be required by the receiving country, which adds additional planning and expense to the exporters. Although the World Organisation for Animal Health (formerly Office International des Epizooties [OIE]) removed VS from its list of internationally reportable diseases in 2015, the United States remains bound by most bilateral trade agreements with its trade partners to immediately report the occurrence of VS and provide information on response measures and updates on the outbreak.

HISTORY AND MANAGEMENT OF THE DISEASE IN THE UNITED STATES

During the past 20 years, VS outbreaks in the United States have been geographically confined mainly to the southwestern and Rocky Mountain regions of the country and have primarily involved the VSNJV serotype of the virus. Large multiyear outbreaks have been temporally separated in 4 to 8-year increments with smaller, single incursion outbreak years occurring sporadically in between. A summary of outbreak years, affected states, virus serotype, and number of affected livestock premises during this time period is presented in **Table 1**. Historically, equine premises make up the majority of the affected premises identified during each outbreak year, although affected cattle

Table 1 Summary of VS outbreaks in the United States within the past 20 y including outbreak year, affected states, virus serotype, and number of affected livestock premises				
Outbreak Year	Number of States Affected	States	VSV Serotype	Number of Affected Premises
2004	3	CO, NM, and TX	VSNJV	294
2005	9	AZ, CO, ID, MT, NE, NM, TX, UT, and WY	VSNJV	445
2006	1	WY	VSNJV	13
2009	2	NM and TX	VSNJV	5
2010	1	AZ	VSNJV	2
2012	2	CO and NM	VSNJV	36
2014	4	AZ, CO, NE, and TX	VSNJV	435
2015	8	AZ, CO, NE, NM, SD, TX, UT, and WY	VSNJV	823
2019	8	CO, KS, NE, NM, OK, TX, UT, and WY	VSIV	1144
2020	8	AR, AZ, KS, MO, NE, NM, OK, and TX	VSIV and VSNJV (TX)	326

Abbreviations: AR, Arkansas; AZ, Arizona; CO, Colorado; ID, Idaho; KS, Kansas; MO, Missouri; MT, Montana; NE, Nebraska; NM, New Mexico; OK, Oklahoma; SD, South Dakota; TX, Texas; UT, Utah; WY, Wyoming.

premises are also routinely documented, especially during large outbreaks. Several factors may be involved in why equine premises are more frequently affected during an outbreak, such as vector preference for equids and/or common management practices on equine premises. For example, daily feeding and handling practices on equine premises make it more likely that clinically affected horses will be noticed by owners or barn managers, as opposed to grazing cattle operations where the animals may not be observed directly for days or weeks at a time and even when observed may not be noticed to have a clinical abnormality. In the Rocky Mountain region of the United States, many beef cattle herds are moved to high mountain pastures for the summer months and will not be physically observed until gathered again in the fall. Equine owners are also more likely to seek veterinary care in response to noticing a clinical abnormality in their horse. Increased biosecurity and intensive management on dairy farms can have a protective effect; however when dairy cattle become VSV-infected, significant short-term production losses often result both from reduced feed intake in cows with oral lesions and inability to milk cows with painful teat or udder lesions.

Ongoing surveillance for FMD and other foreign vesicular diseases of concern in the United States requires that USDA-accredited private veterinarians immediately report to state and federal animal health officials on suspected vesicular lesion occurrence in all livestock species. Follow-up on each report is conducted by a local state or federal veterinary medical officer specifically trained as a foreign animal disease diagnostician who deploys to the affected livestock premises, examines the animals, collects the appropriate diagnostic samples, and places a quarantine on the premises as designated by authority of the state animal health official (SAHO). Diagnostic samples are shipped overnight to the USDA's National Veterinary Services Laboratories (NVSL) in either Ames, Iowa, or Plum Island, New York, depending on the species affected. Samples from vesicular lesioned equids, which cannot be affected with FMD, go to NVSL in Ames, Iowa, with diagnostic testing for VS as the primary rule out, whereas samples from lesioned ruminants and swine go to NVSL on Plum Island for primary rule out of FMD and foreign swine vesicular diseases, followed by secondary rule out of VS, and tertiary testing for domestic vesicular diseases, such as bluetongue, epizootic hemorrhagic disease, and bovine papular stomatitis in cattle and Senecavirus A in swine.

In all suspect cases, samples to be collected from lesioned animals include a serum sample and swabs of the lesions submitted in viral transport media. Diagnostic assays at NVSL used to confirm VSV-infection are specific to each VSV serotype and include antibody detection methods on serum samples, such as competitive enzyme-linked immunosorbent assay (cELISA), complement fixation test (CFT), virus neutralization, and virus detection methods on swab samples, such as real-time reverse transcription polymerase chain reaction (rRT-PCR) and virus isolation (VI). Although the cELISA provides an early indication of recent infection and will test positive a few days prior to the CFT in a naïve, recently exposed animal, the cELISA may subsequently remain positive for up to 10 to 12 years.[17] Given the number of previously exposed livestock residing in historically affected regions in the United States, the cELISA alone cannot be used to confirm recent infection unless occurring in an animal that was either not geographically present in a previous outbreak region or in an animal too young to have experienced the last US outbreak. The CFT, rRT-PCR, and/or VI are used as reliable indicators of recent infection for the purposes of VS case definition during an outbreak. All case definitions for VS require compatible clinical signs and have several options for diagnostic confirmation using these assays. An immunoglobulin M capture ELISA has been developed recently at NVSL and may also be used as a reliable indicator of recent infection in future outbreaks. Although the VS index case for the nation, index cases for newly affected states, and VS cases in ruminants and swine require diagnostic confirmation at NVSL, since 2015, the USDA-approved National Animal Health Laboratory Network laboratories located in historically VS-affected states have been activated during outbreaks to conduct VSV testing in clinically affected equids. This action has successfully increased laboratory capacity and reduced result turnaround time during an outbreak response.

Once an index case of VS is diagnostically confirmed in the United States, a national situation report is issued first to state and federal animal health officials and bilateral trade partners for their awareness, and then the report is publicly posted to the USDA-APHIS website.[2] At least once-weekly situation reports are issued and posted throughout the outbreak thereafter until the incident is declared over, usually 30 days after the last quarantine release in the country. A joint state–federal response following standardized response protocols and using local personnel is organized in each affected state. A national-level situation unit leader is activated to provide support, maintain response continuity across states, gather data, and issue situation reports. SAHOs provide electronic communication by mass email to private veterinarians licensed to practice in the state notifying them of the confirmation of a VS case, recommending increased surveillance and educational outreach to clients, reminding of reporting requirements, and providing instructions on response measures. Information is also posted to SAHOs' websites, including specifics of any new interstate movement and entry requirements enacted as a response measure.

Livestock premises with laboratory diagnostic results meeting a VS confirmed case definition are categorized as confirmed positive premises. Once a county is confirmed as VSV-positive, new equine premises presenting with clinical signs of VSV in that county are not required to be tested for confirmation of the disease but the premises is quarantined and classified as a suspect premises. All clinical cases in ruminants or swine are required to be tested regardless of their presence in an already confirmed infected county. Premises may additionally be classified as suspect if clinical animals on the premises fail to meet a confirmed case definition but have diagnostic evidence of recent VSV infection. All confirmed positive and suspect VS premises are placed under state quarantine for a minimum of 14 days from the onset of lesions in the last affected animal on the premises. The quarantine applies to all VS-susceptible species on the premises and no movement of these species off-site is permitted without the approval of the state veterinarian.

Isolation of lesioned animals from nonlesioned animals is instituted to reduce spread of the virus by direct contact, and aggressive vector control recommendations are provided to be instituted by the premises/animal owner to further reduce within-herd spread. Oversight of equine premises is conducted by private veterinarians communicating with SAHOs in most states, whereas oversight of ruminant and swine premises is conducted directly by state or federal animal health officials. Private veterinarians or animal health officials overseeing each premises confirm the 14-day countdown after the onset of lesions in the last affected animal. SAHOs issue a quarantine release once this time period has passed with no new cases presenting. Continuation of aggressive vector control on the premises is recommended throughout the remainder of the outbreak because reinfection of previously affected animals and lesion-development in new animals after quarantine release has occurred occasionally from continued presence of infected vectors in the general area when vector mitigations on the premises are inadequate.

DISCUSSION

Recent outbreaks of VS in the United States have provided evidence that climate change may be affecting the future size, scope, and geographic range of outbreaks.

The 2019 and 2020 VS outbreaks shared some characteristic features of historic outbreaks in the United States but also had several unexpected attributes potentially related to climatic factors. The 2019 VSIV outbreak resulted in the identification of 1144 VSV-affected premises in 111 counties in 8 states. The factors that magnified this outbreak to become the largest in both size and geographic scope in the past 40 years are still a relative mystery, although climatological and ecological conditions affecting vector abundance, dispersal, or habitat quality are suspected to be involved. Indeed, the previous round of outbreaks in 2014 to 2015 was also larger than normal by comparison to other years and may hold the key to the identification of climatic factors that may have been intensifying into 2019. Questions remain regarding what caused US outbreaks to be dominated exclusively by the VSNJV serotype since the last VSIV outbreak in 1997 to 1998 and, subsequently, what changed that allowed VSIV to appear and surge alone so successfully in 2019. Clinically, the VSNJV and VSIV presented across the outbreaks quite similarly with the full gamut of lesion types represented and neither virus serotype looking any more or less virulent in the animals than the other.

Phylogenetic analysis supports the occurrence of an overwintering event of VSIV between the 2019 and 2020 outbreaks.[18] Although overwintering of the virus was an expected event based on historic occurrences of the same, there were several completely unexpected outcomes that followed. Based on study of the 2004 to 2006 and 2014 to 2015 outbreaks and the dynamics previously described on incursion years versus expansion years, the 2020 outbreak was expected to begin with new cases in all the same states where last observed in 2019 and then expand outward from those saturated regions. It began as predicted with the first cases of 2020 identified early in the season and in previously affected areas in the lower southwestern states before expanding northward, apparently mirroring expected temporal peaks of vector abundance. However, the expected cases in the Rocky Mountain states (Colorado, Utah, and Wyoming) were never observed. This region with the most cases in 2019 had zero cases confirmed in 2020 despite strong surveillance and testing. It is known that this outcome is not due to an immunity to the virus by the previously exposed animals. High antibody titers to VSV from previous outbreak years have failed to prevent individual animals from developing lesions in the next outbreak year. Anecdotally, horse owners in historically affected VS-regions have reported that the same horse or horses in their herd developed lesions during every outbreak since living there. Additionally, several animals in each outbreak are typically identified with new lesions after the previous lesions have healed on premises where the vector control is determined to have been inadequate. These cases suggest no resistance to infected vector reexposure with the same virus, despite very high antibody titers, which necessitates the premises be requarantined and a more aggressive vector control program administered. There were 5 such cases documented during the 2019 to 2020 outbreak.

One hypothesis for the 2020 absence of VS cases in the Rocky Mountain region is that the environmental conditions in the area did not support the high-volume of black flies and *Culicoides* spp that were present in 2019. Specifically, Colorado, Utah, and Wyoming were experiencing extreme drought conditions throughout 2020, which may have affected the vector hatch and overall insect populations. Further in-depth study is planned to evaluate this hypothesis and investigate other potential causes.

Another unexpected outcome in the 2020 outbreak was the development of a new outbreak region in the Kansas/Missouri/Oklahoma/Arkansas area. Although Kansas and Oklahoma each confirmed a single VSV-infected premises in 2019 in counties bordering active VSV-infected states, neither state had previously reported cases in at least the past 50 years. Kansas and Oklahoma were anticipated to identify more cases in 2020 in western portions of the states where 2019 cases were found but, instead, the 2020 outbreak erupted far to the east in both states and spilled over into western Missouri and northwest Arkansas. More study is needed to evaluate how the virus moved and flourished farther east than expected.

Finally, there was a new 2020 incursion of a VSNJV serotype virus in south Texas during the ongoing VSIV outbreak occurring in the western part of the state hundreds of miles away, which is a rare dynamic last observed in the 1997 to 1998 outbreak and has never been fully explained. It is unknown what if any VS cases were occurring on the other side of the border in Mexico at the same time, which could provide better insight to the situation. Full genomic sequencing and phylogenetic analysis are planned to investigate the potential origin of both viruses and the relationship of the 2019 and 2020 isolates to viruses circulating more recently in Mexico. All of these unusual occurrences during the 2019 and 2020 outbreaks may be indicators of changes in climatic and environmental factors inducing a noticeable shift in the epidemiology of a historically observed vector-borne disease.

SUMMARY

VS is a vector-borne livestock disease caused either by VSNJV or by VSIV. The disease circulates endemically in northern South America, Central America, and Mexico and only occasionally causes outbreaks in the United States. Veterinarians are required to report suspected cases to state and federal animal health officials. During the past 20 years, VS outbreaks in the southwestern and Rocky Mountain regions occurred periodically with incursion years followed by virus overwintering and subsequent expansion outbreak years. Regulatory response by animal health officials prevents spread from lesioned animals and manages trade impacts. Private veterinary practitioners play a significant role during VS outbreaks through initial identification and reporting of cases, diagnostic sample collection and submission, management of lesioned animals, assisting in premises quarantine countdowns and releases, and advising animal owners on biosecurity and vector mitigation procedures. VSV is a zoonotic pathogen, which can be transmitted to humans through direct contact with lesioned animals and which results in flu-like symptoms. Personal protective equipment and good biosecurity practices should be used by veterinarians and animal handlers when handling livestock with active VS lesions. Recent US outbreaks of VS highlight potential climate change impacts on insect vectors or other transmission-related variables that may result in shifting epidemiology of the disease in future outbreak years.

CLINICS CARE POINTS

- VS is a disease reportable to state and federal animal health officials in the United States. Veterinarians suspecting VS in a clinical animal should contact either the State Veterinarian or the federal Area Veterinarian in Charge (AVIC) for the state in which the animal is located.

- Diagnostic samples to collect in suspect VS cases include a serum sample and swabs of the lesions in viral transport media. Samples must be submitted to a USDA-approved VSV laboratory with the authorization of the State Veterinarian or federal AVIC.

- VS is a self-limiting disease and the lesions in most affected livestock heal within a couple of weeks without veterinary intervention; however, some older animals or those with underlying health conditions may require supportive care, especially in cases with severe oral lesions where the animals cease to eat or drink.

- Isolation of lesioned animals and implementation of aggressive vector control measures is imperative to reduce the spread of VSV during an outbreak.

- VSV is a zoonotic pathogen, which can be transmitted to humans through direct contact with lesioned animals. Personal protective equipment and good biosecurity practices should be used by veterinarians and animal handlers when handling livestock with active VS lesions.

DISCLOSURE

The author has nothing to disclose.

REFERENCES

1. Rodriguez LL. Emergence and Re-Emergence of Vesicular Stomatitis in the United States. Virus Res 2002;85:211–9.
2. Vesicular Stomatitis Outbreak Situation Reports on USDA-APHIS. Available at: https://www.aphis.usda.gov/aphis/ourfocus/animalhealth/animal-disease-information/cattle-disease-information/vesicular-stomatitis-info. [Accessed 11 June 2022].
3. Pelzel-McCluskey AM. Vesicular Stomatitis. Available at:. In: Winter AL, editor. Merck veterinary manual. online edition. Kenilworth, NJ, USA: Merck & Co, Inc.; 2020 https://www.merckvetmanual.com/generalized-conditions/vesicular-stomatitis/vesicular-stomatitis-in-large-animals. [Accessed 11 June 2022].
4. Duarte PC, Morley PS, Traub-Dargatz JL, et al. Factors Associated with Vesicular Stomatitis in Animals in the Western United States. J Am Vet Med Assoc 2008; 232:249–56.
5. Mohler JR. Vesicular stomatitis of horses and cattle; Bulletin No 662. Washington, DC, USA: United States Department of Agriculture; 1918.
6. Hanson RP. The natural history of vesicular stomatitis. Bacteriol Rev 1952;16: 179–204.
7. Schmidtmann ET, Tabachnick WJ, Hunt GJ, et al. 1995 Epizootic of Vesicular Stomatitis (New Jersey Serotype) in the Western United States: An Entomologic Perspective. J Med Entomol 1999;36:1–7.
8. Tesh RB, Boshell SJ, Modi GB, et al. Natural Infection of Humans, Animals, and Phlebotomine Sand Flies with the Alagoas Serotype of Vesicular Stomatitis Virus in Colombia. Am J Trop Med Hyg 1987;36:653–61.
9. Schnitzlein W, Reichmann M. Characterization of New Jersey Vesicular Stomatitis Virus Isolates from Horses and Black Flies during the 1982 Outbreak in Colorado. Virology 1985;142:426–31.
10. Elias E, McVey DS, Peters D, et al. Contributions of Hydrology to Vesicular Stomatitis Virus Emergence in the Western USA. Ecosystems 2018;22:416–33.
11. Rainwater-Lovett K, Pauszek SJ, Kelley WN, et al. Molecular Epidemiology of Vesicular Stomatitis New Jersey Virus from the 2004–2005 US Outbreak Indicates a Common Origin with Mexican Strains. J Gen Virol 2007;88:2042–51.
12. Rodriguez LL, Bunch TA, Fraire M, et al. Re-Emergence of Vesicular Stomatitis in the Western United States Is Associated with Distinct Viral Genetic Lineages. Virology 2000;271:171–81.
13. Velazquez-Salinas L, Pauszek SJ, Zarate S, et al. Phylogeographic Characteristics of Vesicular Stomatitis New Jersey Viruses Circulating in Mexico from 2005

to 2011 and Their Relationship to Epidemics in the United States. Virology 2014; 449:17–24.

14. Mason, J.; Herrera Saldaña, A.; Turner, W.J. Vesicular Stomatitis in Mexico. In Proceedings of the Annual Meeting of the United States Animal Health Association, Miami Beach, FL, USA, 7–12 November 1976;Volume 80, pp. 234–253.

15. Peters DPC, McVey DS, Elias EH, et al. Big Data-Model Integration and AI for Vector-Borne Disease Prediction. Ecosphere 2020;11:e03157.

16. Pelzel-McCluskey AM. Economic impacts of vesicular stomatitis outbreaks. Equine Dis Q 2015;24:5.

17. Toms, D; Powell, M; Redlinger, M; Beach, T; Jenkins-Moore, et al. Monitoring of Four Naturally Infected Horses for Vesicular Stomatitis Antibody. In Proceedings of the Annual Meeting American Association of Veterinary Laboratory Diagnosticians, Greensboro, NC, USA, 2012. Available at: https://www.aavld.org/assets/2012_AnnualMeeting/Proceedings/97280%20aavld12_progabs.proceeding.book.pdf (accessed on 28 June 2022).

18. Pelzel-McCluskey AM, Christensen B, Humphreys J, et al. Review of Vesicular Stomatitis in the United States with Focus on 2019 and 2020 Outbreaks. Pathogens 2021;10:993.

Lumpy Skin Disease

Alessandra Di Giuseppe, DVM[a],*, Valentina Zenobio, DVM[b],
Francesca Dall'Acqua, BSc (Zoology), MSc (Veterinary Epidemiology)[b],
Daria Di Sabatino, DVM[b], Paolo Calistri, DVM[b]

KEYWORDS

- Lumpy skin disease (LSD) • Vector-borne disease • Transboundary • Cattle
- Skin nodules • Clinics

KEY POINTS

- Lumpy skin disease (LSD) is a contagious non-zoonotic viral disease of cattle.
- Susceptible hosts contract the virus principally by mechanical means from hematophagous arthropods, including biting flies, mosquitoes, and ticks.
- Principal clinical signs are fever (>41°C), subscapular and prefemoral lymph node enlargement, nodular skin lesions (10–50 mm), edema of the limbs, and ocular and nasal discharge.
- LSD is a threat to livestock health and food security, especially in lower income countries.
- The disease is of great concern due to the recent rapid spread in free countries and the potential impact of direct and indirect economic damages.

INTRODUCTION

Lumpy skin disease (LSD) is a contagious non-zoonotic viral disease of cattle. It is caused by LSD virus (LSDV) for which the Neethling strain is the prototype.[1]

LSDV, a double-stranded DNA virus, belongs to the genus *Capripoxvirus* of the family Poxviridae along with goatpox virus (GTPV) and sheeppox virus (SPPV). LSDV shares strong antigenic relationship with SPPV and GTPV, and its genome is approximately 151 kbp and with 156 genes.[2]

LSDV is very resistant to inactivation, surviving in necrotic skin nodules for up to 33 days or longer, desiccated crusts for up to 35 days, and at least 18 days in air-dried hides. The virus is susceptible to sunlight and detergents containing lipid solvents, but in dark environmental conditions, such as contaminated animal sheds, it

---

[a] Veterinary Operations Center for Epidemiology, Programming, Information (COVEPI), Istituto Zooprofilattico dell'Abruzzo e del Molise "G. Caporale" or Experimental Zooprophylactic Institute of Abruzzo and Molise "G. Caporale", Teramo, Italy; [b] Istituto Zooprofilattico Sperimentaledell'Abruzzo e del Molise "G. Caporale", Teramo, Italy
* Corresponding author. Istituto Zooprofilattico Sperimentaledell'Abruzzo e del Molise "G. Caporale", via Campo Boario | 64100 TERAMO | ITALIA
E-mail address: a.digiuseppe@izs.it

can persist for many months. LSDV is killed at 55°C for 2 hours and 65°C for 30 minutes; it can be recovered from skin nodules kept at −80°C for 10 years and infected tissue culture fluid stored at 4°C for 6 months.[2]

Globalization, which has made changes in trading patterns of animals and animal products, global climate change and civil conflicts occurring in some countries, has aided the continuous spread of LSDV. LSD is a threat to livestock health and food security, especially in lower income countries. These threats include important production losses, loss of draught power, trade restrictions, and long-term convalescence. For this reason, it is listed as a notifiable disease in bovines by the World Organisation for Animal Health (WOAH).[3] It has never been found in the United States nor in North America,[4] but because of these risks and the high consequences of the disease, LSD is a US Department of Agriculture (USDA) Animal and Plant Health Inspection Service notifiable disease and also on the USDA select agent list.[5]

These characteristics of the disease and several factors related to its evolving epidemiology raise a great concern in terms of introduction and difficulty of eradication, that is (1) nonstop and rapid spread toward Southeast Asia, (2) reoccurrence in countries where control and preventive measures had achieved eradication, such as Russia, (3) endemicity in previously free countries, such as Turkey, and (4) spread to regions experiencing a colder climate.[6]

If an outbreak of LSD was to occur in the United States or North America, there could be several consequences, including.

1. *Economic Impact:* The disease can result in significant economic losses due to reduced milk and meat production, as well as potential trade restrictions on affected animals and animal products. The US cattle industry is a major component of the agricultural economy, and any disruption could have widespread economic consequences.
2. *Trade Restrictions:* The appearance of LSD may lead to trade restrictions imposed by other countries to prevent the spread of the virus. This can impact international trade in cattle, beef, and other related products.
3. *Livestock Health:* The disease could affect the health of livestock, leading to increased mortality rates and decreased productivity. This, in turn, could have cascading effects on the overall agricultural sector and food supply.
4. *Control Measures:* Controlling the spread of LSD would require significant resources and efforts. This may include culling infected animals, implementing quarantine measures, and conducting vaccination campaigns.
5. *Public Perception:* The presence of a contagious livestock disease could lead to concerns among the public regarding food safety and animal health. This may result in increased scrutiny of agricultural practices and potentially impact consumer confidence.
6. *Wildlife Impact:* Although LSD primarily affects cattle, there could be concerns about the potential impact on wildlife. Understanding and managing the disease in both domestic and wild animal populations would be essential.
7. *Collaboration and Research:* An outbreak may prompt increased collaboration between government agencies, researchers, and the agricultural industry to understand the dynamics of the disease, develop effective control measures, and prevent further spread.

It is important to note that these consequences would depend on various factors, including the spread and degree of the outbreak, the effectiveness of control measures implemented, and the response from both the government and the agricultural community. Early detection and rapid reaction well-coordinated responses are crucial in mitigating the impact of such diseases.

EPIDEMIOLOGY
Hosts and Transmission of Lumpy Skin Disease Virus

The severity of the clinical signs of LSD is highly variable and depends on a number of factors, including the strain of the virus, the age of the host, its immunologic status, and the breed of the host. LSD is host-specific; *Bos taurus* is generally more susceptible to clinical disease than *Bos indicus* and Asian buffaloes (*Bubalus* spp). Indeed, the morbidity rate is significantly lower in buffalo (1.6%) than in cattle (30.8%).[7]

Within *B taurus*, the fine-skinned Channel Island breeds develop more severe disease, with lactating cows appearing to be most at risk. However, even among groups of cattle of the same breed kept together under the same conditions, there is a large variation in the clinical signs presented, ranging from subclinical infection to death.[8] There may be failure of the virus to infect the whole group, probably depending on the virulence of the virus, immunologic status of the host, host genotype, and vector prevalence.[3]

LSDV infection has also been reported in animals other than cattle. Specifically, these animals were mainly free-ranging African buffaloes (*Syncerus caffer*) (Kenya, 1981; South Africa, 2014) and the Asian water buffalo (*Bubalus bubalis*) (India, 2020; Egypt, 2016–2019 the buffalo species was not specified) and were found to be serologically positive. Antibodies against capripox viruses were detected also in other African wild ruminant species like Arabian Oryx (*Oryx leucoryx*) in a wildlife reserve in Saudi Arabia (1989), in southern elands (*Taurotragus oryx*) in Namibia (2019), and in Springboks (*Antidorcas marsupialis*), Impalas (*Aepyceros melampus*), and wildebeests (*Connochaetes gnou, C taurinus*) in South Africa (1933–1995).[9] In addition, southern eland (*T oryx*) was also reported positive to LSDV by polymerase chain reaction (PCR) in Namibia (2019). A captive giraffe (*Giraffa camelopardalis*) resulted positive to LSDV by PCR and virus isolation in a zoo of a large city in northern Vietnam in 2021.[6] It seems that *Stomoxys calcitrans* (stable fly) is the most competent vector of LSDV, as well as the mosquito species *Aedes aegypti*.

Being cosmopolite, *S calcitrans* might have a greater worldwide impact than previously thought on animal and human pathogen transmission.[10]

Ae aegypti (Linnaeus, 1762) is one of the most prolific mosquito vector species in the world. It is found on every continent—except the Antarctic—and has played major roles in various vector-borne disease outbreaks over the last century.

Future climate change will affect *Ae aegypti* distribution and will surely have major impacts on public health decision-making across the globe. In future climate change scenarios, the northern hemisphere will have extended *Ae aegypti* distribution, whereas the southern hemisphere will have the opposite outcomes.

Europe will become more suitable for *Ae aegypti* and its related vector-borne diseases. The loss of suitability in the Brazilian Amazon region further indicated that this tropical rainforest biome will have lower levels of precipitation to support this species in the future.[11]

By contrast, *Culicoides nubeculosus* (biting midges), *Anopheles stephensi*, and *Culex quinquefasciatus* (mosquitoes) are likely to be inefficient vectors of LSDV.[12–14] It is suggested that horseflies, as *Haematopota* spp and *Tabanus bromiums,* could be more effective in transmitting the virus than the stable fly and albeit nonbiting flies as *Musca domestica* and *Muscina stabulans* could be LSDV carriers.

The Tabanidae have a worldwide distribution. Species of *Tabanus* and *Chrysops* are found in temperate and tropical areas, but *Haematopota* is absent from South America and Australasia and is uncommon in North America.[15]

LSDV was isolated from hard ticks such as *Dermacentor marginatus, Hyalomma asiaticum, Rhipicephalus appendiculatus, R Boophilus, Amblyomma hebraeum,* and

Hyalomma truncatum. Moreover, intrastadial transmission and transtadial persistence of the virus was demonstrated by *A hebraeum and R appendiculatus* ticks, which may play an important role in the transmission of LSDV. Moreover, transovarial passage occurred in *Rhipicephalus annulatus,* and the virus could persist through the winter in *A hebraeum* nymphs and *R decoloratus*, implying that these ticks might serve as a reservoir for LSDV.[6] The transmission of LSDV via direct contact between animals is considered to be inefficient. Once infected, animals exhibit clinical symptoms and they begin to release the virus in their saliva, as well as through ocular and nasal discharges, thereby contaminating shared feeding and drinking troughs.[16,17] Bull semen is shown to be a possible route of infection. Moreover, in one study that tested an LSD-infected herd, neutralizing antibodies were detected in a 1-day old calf, providing evidence of intrauterine transmission.[17] Sucking calves may get infected via milk or from skin lesions in the teats (rare due to maternal antibodies).[16] In addition, based on one single study, the transmission through bovine meat and offal products would be very low.[16] Iatrogenic transmission may occur (eg, using the same needle for multiple animals).

Following experimental infection, it seemed that lymph nodes and testicles of clinically and subclinically infected animals were reservoirs of live LSDV, whereas live virus was not detected in deep skeletal meat.[6]

Risk Factors

The main risk factors of LSD spread are associated with the introduction of the virus through blood-feeding insects (spread occurs at short distances) and through legal or illegal animal movements (spread can occur at long distances).[6] In low-income or politically unstable countries, the lack of control of transboundary animal movements may favor the illegal or uncontrolled movement of potentially infected cattle.

Cattle density, higher temperatures, and rainfall correlated with a higher vector activity should be considered factors able to increase the risk of outbreaks.[6] In Ethiopia, communal grazing and watering points were found to be associated with the occurrence of LSD.[18]

Novel live vaccine-like strains most likely originated from a poorly manufactured Lumpivax vaccine (KEVEVAPI), and these strains have emerged and were responsible for some LSD outbreaks in Russia and China,[19] raising on one hand the need for implementing regulatory measures concerning vaccine manufacturing and on the other highlighting how poor quality vaccines can serve as risk factors for LSD introduction.

In the United States and North America, the identification of hotspots for the risk of introduction, based on illegal animal movement patterns or on the distribution of harbors and other sites of animal import, can ensure targeted surveillance and control measures with the best use of available resources.

World-Wide Morbidity and Mortality Rates

The morbidity rates in LSD epidemics vary enormously, ranging from 2% to 45%.[20] The high variation of intra-herd morbidity and the high rates in many farms are most likely linked to the small size of the affected farms.[21] The overall morbidity observed in Serbia in 2016 was 13.6% and up to 9% in Israel in 2019.[22] Mortality due to LSD varies between 1% and 3%, but up to 40% has been reported in severe outbreak situations.[23] These broad ranges for morbidity and mortality are likely to be due to variations in cattle breed, health status, viral strain, and insect vectors involved in the transmission.

Geographic Distribution

LSD was first reported in Zambia in 1929; 15 years later, it was observed in Botswana and then in South Africa, where 8 million cattle were affected by the disease.[3]

The disease subsequently spread northwards, becoming endemic in most sub-Saharan areas.[23]

In 1989, for the first time, the disease spread out of the African continent into Israel[24] and from there further into the Middle East region. According to the WOAH, LSD was reported in Kuwait in 1991, Lebanon in 1993, Yemen in 1995, United Arab Emirates in 2000, Bahrain in 2003, Israel in 2006 to 2007, and Oman in 2010.[25] Since 2012, LSD has been spreading on a scale never observed before, reaching Turkey, an important crossroad between Asia and Europe. The year after, LSD was also reported in Jordan, Iraq, Palestinian Autonomous Territories, Azerbaijan, Iran, and Kuwait.[25]

In 2015, LSD was observed for the first time in Europe. During that year, Greece reported 111 outbreaks close to the border with Turkey. In the same year, Russia experienced for the first time an LSD epidemic near the border with Azerbaijan.[25]

Saudi Arabia was affected in June 2015,[25] and in the following years, the infection spread across the Balkan region (Albania, Bulgaria, Montenegro, North Macedonia, and Serbia) and was detected in Georgia and Kazakhstan.[25] Thanks to the multicountry mass vaccination campaign with homologous LSD vaccine, Balkan countries succeeded in containing the disease, which has not been reported in the area after 2017.[22] Following the first detection in the Russian Federation in 2015, LSD spread to several Asian countries: Kazakhstan, China, Nepal, Pakistan, India, Bhutan, Vietnam, Thailand, Myanmar, Sri Lanka, Malaysia, Laos, and Taiwan, eventually reaching Mongolia and Eastern Siberia. In 2022 to 2023, 3 countries reported the disease for the first time: Afghanistan, Indonesia, and Libya. Moreover, in 2023, LSD reoccurred in the south of Israel at the border with the Gaza strip.[3,25] The United States and North America are disease free.

Given the potential for the rapid spread of LSD through blood-feeding insects and movements of animals, it is crucial for the United States and North America to remain vigilant. Some specific considerations include.

1. *Surveillance and Early Detection:* Implementing robust surveillance systems to monitor the health of livestock is crucial. Early detection of any signs of LSD can enable swift response measures to prevent further spread.
2. *Quarantine and Control Measures:* Establishing effective quarantine measures in case of an outbreak is essential. This includes restricting the movement of infected animals and implementing control measures to contain the spread of the virus.
3. *Biosecurity Measures:* Enhancing biosecurity measures on farms and in the livestock industry can help prevent the introduction and spread of the disease. This includes measures to control insect vectors, monitoring animal movements and ensuring proper hygiene practices.
4. *Public Awareness and Education:* Raising awareness among farmers, veterinarians, and the general public about the signs of LSD and the importance of reporting any suspicious cases can contribute to early detection and control.
5. *International Cooperation:* Given that legal or illegal animal movements can contribute to the spread of the disease over long distances, cooperation with neighboring countries and international organizations is crucial. Sharing information and collaborating on control measures can help mitigate the risk of cross-border transmission.
6. *Vaccination Programs:* Implementing vaccination programs for livestock in countries where approved can be a proactive measure to build immunity and reduce the impact of the disease.

7. *Research and Preparedness:* Investing in research on the virus, its vectors, and effective control strategies can contribute to better preparedness. This includes having contingency plans in place for responding to potential outbreaks.

By remaining alert, implementing preventive measures, and having effective response strategies in place, the United States and North America can better protect their livestock industry and minimize the potential consequences of an LSD outbreak.

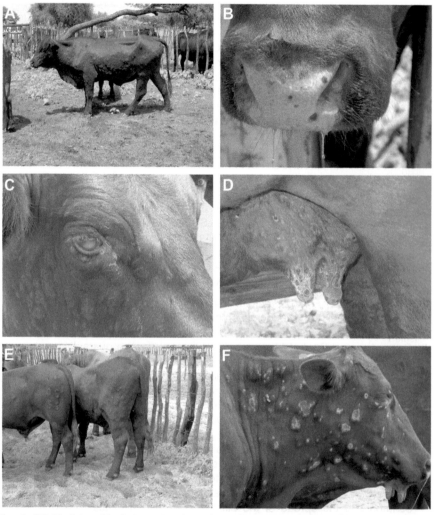

Fig. 1. (*A*) Nodular skin lesions, head, neck, perineum, genitalia, udder, and limbs are preferred places. (*B*) Ulcerative lesions develop in the mucosal surface of the nasal cavities, resulting in a nasal discharge. (*C*) Ulcerative lesions in one or both eyes' corneas can cause blindness. (*D*) The infected nodules on the udder, resulting in the loss of animal productivity for several months. (*E*) Edema of the limbs. (*F*) The infected nodules begin to ulcerate, which may further inflict damage to the leather. (*Data from* Dr. Massimo Scacchia, (IZSAM, Italy), Biewenga farm, Gobabis disctrit, Namibia, 2009.)

CLINICAL OUTCOMES

In the natural host, the incubation period varies between 7 and 28 days. The course of the disease can be acute, subacute, or chronic. The virus replicates in fibroblasts, macrophages, pericytes, and endothelial cells, and the viremia can later cause vasculitis and lymphangitis in infected tissues. Kumar and colleagues[26] stated that the duration of LSD viremia varied from 1 to 10 days. LSDV exhibits a wide tissue tropism, but the preferred sites are the skin on the neck, head, limbs, perineum, udder, and genitalia.[27]

Clinical symptoms (**Table 1**) that appear after the incubation period can be grouped into 4 phases.

The acute phase, in which animals show symptoms of high fever of 41°C or greater, which occurs for 7 to 10 days and is followed by other symptoms such as anorexia, lacrimation, depression, increased nasal discharge, decreased milk production, increased saliva secretion, and multinodular lesions found around the skin and mucous membranes.[28] During the initial days of viral infection, the nodules internally appear grayish-white and may exude serum. However, following disease progression (14 days), the nodules may develop a cone-shaped central core or sequestrum of necrotic material called the "sit-fast."[29] After 1 to 2 days, the nodules burst and are able to spread the virus to the surrounding environment.[28]

The second phase is swelling of the subscapular and precrural lymph nodes as well as an increase in multiple nodules with a diameter of 0.5 to 5 cm, which mostly occur in the head, neck, trunk, genitals, udder, mucous membranes, nasal cavity, and mouth.[28] LSDV localizes in the cutaneous tissue and then causes nodules to develop in skin lesions, which are well circumscribed and range between 2 and 7 cm of diameter. The lesions appear solid with flat-topped papules and nodules and multiple coalescing centers.[30]

In the third phase, 2 to 3 weeks from the beginning of symptoms, nodules ulcerate and necrose. In seriously affected cattle, ulcerative lesions develop in the mucosal surface of the eye and in oral/nasal cavities, resulting in prolonged mastication,

Table 1
Clinical symptoms that appear in the four phases during lumpy skin disease

Clinical Phase	Clinical Signs Include
First phase (acute)	Lachrymation and nasal discharge are first seen. Subscapular and prefemoral lymph nodes are swollen. Fever may last a week (>41 C)
Second phase	Nodular skin lesions (10–50 mm) Infected animals develop numerous lesions. Head, neck, perineum, genitalia, udder, and limbs are preferred places (**Fig. 1**A, D) Edema of the limbs, followed by lesions on the legs and joints, which can cause subcutaneous infections, secondary bacterial infections, and lameness (**Fig. 1**E)
Third phase	Ulcerative lesions in one or both eyes can cause blindness (**Fig. 1**C) Ulcerative lesions develop in the mucosal surface of the eye and in oral/nasal cavities, resulting in prolonged mastication, lacrimation, and nasal discharge (**Fig. 1**B) Deep nodules involve skin, subcutaneous tissue, and occasionally muscles. Necrotic plaques in the oral and nasal mucous membranes induce purulent nasal discharge and excessive salivation. After lesion centers ulcerate and scab over, nodules might last month (**Fig. 1**F)

lacrimation, and nasal discharge.[28,31] As soon as the infected nodules on the mouth, nose, eyes, udder, genitalia, and rectum begin to ulcerate, many cattle suffer from significant emaciation and weakness, resulting in the loss of animal productivity for several months, which may further inflict permanent damage to the leather.[32]

The fourth phase, after at least 1 month, is healing of the ulcers, skin thickening, and hyperpigmentation of the lesion.[28]

Animals that overcome the infection show complete clearance of the viral load and do not act as carriers for LSDV.[33]

The oxidation-anti-oxidation imbalance in infected cattle results in a significant rise in the levels of pro-inflammatory cytokines and adverse effects on animal health, as found in the clinical trial by Ahmed and colleagues.[34] This was positively correlated with histopathological outcomes in infected animals, which showed signs of profuse necrosis, mononuclear cell infiltration, intracytoplasmic inclusion bodies, and severe vasculitis. High levels of the metabolite buildup in the heart, liver, and kidney cause hypophosphatemia, which exacerbates the symptoms of hemolytic anemia.[30,35] Cattle affected with LSDV develop pancytopenia, hyperproteinemia, hyperkalemia, hyperchloremia, and reduced creatinine concentrations.[36] Young cows, lactating mothers, and underweight livestock are more vulnerable to infection by LSDV, possibly due to poor or impaired immunity.[31,37] Calves born from infected dams exhibit resistance toward LSDV for nearly 6 months because of the acquired maternal antibodies.[38] Maternal antibodies have been found in the colostrum of vaccinated cows and then detected by serology in calves fed with that colostrum, after 3 days from calving. The levels of detectable antibodies in the serum of calves decreased after day 3 to 38.5% on day 90 and to 0% on days 120 and 150.[39]

Differential Diagnosis

Similar clinical signs have been reported for pseudo-LSD infection caused by bovine herpesvirus 2 (BoHV-2). This is usually a milder clinical condition, resembling only the early stage of LSD. Pseudo-LSD is characterized by superficial skin lesions located mainly on the face, neck, chest, and perineum. Intra-nuclear inclusion bodies and viral syncytia are histopathological characteristics of BoHV-2 infection not seen in LSD.[3]

There are many diseases causing similar signs of LSD. It is important to obtain a definite diagnosis so applicable preventative and control measures can be performed for susceptible herds. LSD can be confused with the diseases listed in **Table 2**.

DIAGNOSIS

LSD is a disease reportable to state and federal animal health officials in the United States. Veterinarians suspecting LSD in a clinical animal should contact either the State Veterinarian or the Federal Area Veterinarian in Charge (AVIC) for the state in which the animal is located.

LSD can be suspected by typical skin lesions, but other diseases must be considered in the differential diagnosis. Laboratory tests are needed to confirm the infection, such as virus isolation and real-time and conventional PCR (Polymerase Chain Reaction). Virus isolation and PCR are the most sensitive methods for detecting the LSDV on the skin. Serologic tests (serum neutralization test, immunodiffusion gel agar, indirect ELISA (Enzyme Linked Immunosorbent Assay), and indirect fluorescent antibody technique) may be used for monitoring infection in non-vaccinated cattle populations.[28,40]

The RT-PCR (Reverse Transcription Polymerase Chain Reaction) test is a simple, sensitive, fast, and reliable method for detecting LSD viral genome in blood and

Table 2
Differential diagnosis to consider in case of lumpy skin disease

Other Differential Diagnosis for Integumentary Lesions	Differential Diagnosis for Mucosal Lesions
Dermatophilosis (*Dermatophilus congolensis*)	Foot and mouth disease
Dermatophytosis	Bluetongue
Photosensitization	Bovine viral diarrhea
Actinomycosis	Malignant catarrhal fever
Actinobacillosis	Infectious bovine rhinotracheitis
Urticaria	Bovine papular stomatitis
Tick bites	
Besnoitiosis	
Nocardiosis ·	
Demodicosis	
Onchocerciasis	
Pseudo-cowpox and cowpox	
Epitheliotropic cutaneous lymphoma and cutaneous lymphoma	

skin nodule biopsies of suspected infected bovines. The samples used to detect LSDV DNA by PCR or RT-PCR methods were skin nodules, secretions, and blood from infected animals. Material for virus isolation and antigen detection should be collected as biopsies or from skin nodules at postmortem examination.[28,40]

Samples for virus isolation should preferably are collected within the first week of the occurrence of clinical signs before the development of neutralizing antibodies. The virus can be isolated from skin nodules for at least 3 to 4 weeks post-infection. For virus isolation, buffy coat from blood collected into heparin or ethylene diamine tetra-acetic acid during the viraemic stage of LSD (before generalization of lesions or within 4 days of generalization) can also be used.[28]

Samples for genome detection using conventional or real-time PCR may be collected when neutralizing antibodies are present. Following the first appearance of the skin lesions, the virus can be isolated for up to 35 days and viral nucleic acid can be demonstrated via PCR for up to 3 months. A quantitative real-time PCR assay has been developed to distinguish the Neethling vaccine strain from the wild-type virus. However, this assay has not proven to be able to distinguish the Neethling strain from some particular field strains such as the novel recombinant LSDV strains from Asia[41] and the LSDV field strains belonging within the cluster 1.1 from South Africa.[42,43]

CONTROL MEASURES, PREVENTION, AND MANAGEMENT

LSD can cause large economic losses due to direct and indirect effects. Although mortality can be quite low, the affected animals suffer from loss of appetite, which can cause a decline in milk production. Nodular lesions are responsible for the decrease in value of hides, which cannot be used for leather production. The ban on movement of animals from infected areas as well as the restrictions posed to the trade of animal products (bodies, skins and semen) adds to the economic losses.

In the majority of cases, the application of one control measure alone is not effective. More often, a combination of control measures must be applied into a well-defined strategy on the basis of the specific epidemiologic situation in that country or region. Moreover, the economic and sociocultural contests are fundamental aspects to be taken into consideration for the success of the eradication strategy.

Vaccination

Vaccination is used to reduce the clinical impact of the disease in animals and to reduce the transmission and spread of wild strains of the virus. Live attenuated heterologous and homologous vaccines have been widely used, both in endemic areas and in free countries during epidemics. Currently, no LSD vaccine has been approved in the United States or North America.

Heterologous vaccines, derived from GTPV and SPPV, are generally used in areas where LSD and GTPV overlap in cattle, sheep, and goats. To achieve a good level of protection in cattle, heterologous vaccines must be administered at a higher dosage than that used in small ruminants. During the epidemic of 2013 in Israel, the heterologous vaccine RM65 SPPV was demonstrated to be less effective than the attenuated homologous Neethling strain LSDV vaccine, even if administered at 10 times the small ruminant dose.[44] In Turkey, the disease is considered endemic.[20] Many vaccination campaigns using the sheep pox strain-based vaccine have been conducted since 2013. Also in Russia, where outbreaks occurred in 2015, and then spread eastward in 2019,[3,25] the SPP vaccine campaign did not succeed in eliminating the virus. Weiss produced the first live attenuated homologous LSD vaccine in 1963 from the Neethling strain in South Africa (Onderstepoort Biological Products).[45]

From that point forward, the Neethling strain was most frequently used in homologous vaccination campaigns. The vaccination campaign put in place in the Balkan regions with a live attenuated homologous strain involved 1.8 million cattle since 2015, and along with other control measures, it was able to stop the epidemic with no outbreaks in the region since 2018 (except for Albania and Montenegro).[3,25]

Both heterologous and homologous vaccines can cause mild side effects, such as swelling at the site of injection, transitory fever, and drop in milk yield. Sometimes, small nodules appear in generalized localizations in the body in vaccinated cattle. Homologous vaccine side effects have been observed in different vaccination campaigns. In Israel, a low percentage (0.5%) of animals vaccinated with the Neethling strain exhibited the so-called Neethling disease,[44] a milder form of LSD that appears for a short period of time (2–3 weeks) after vaccination. In Greece, clinical signs similar to those of LSD and lasting for more than 2 weeks were reported after vaccination.[46,47] In Croatia, the first European country to apply preventive vaccination, only 0.09% of vaccinated animals developed adverse effects.[48]

According to a model of transmission between farms, vaccination is more effective on reducing LSD spread than culling strategies, even when it has a low effectiveness. When 95% of the population is vaccinated, with 75% of the animals effectively protected, total stamping out or partial stamping out have the same probability of eradicating the disease (even if the vaccination is applied between 15 and 65 days after the virus introduction).[29] Preventive vaccination, in the buffer area outside the infected zones, applied to the whole cattle population (no gender and age limitations) succeeded in halting the epidemic in the Balkan Regions, and is to date the strategy provided for by European legislation.[49] In endemic contests (such as the African continent), annual vaccination is recommended in order to impede the reoccurrence of disease between inter-epidemic periods (until 15 years) and take the disease under control. On the other hand, in free periods, LSD becomes a neglected disease and farmers often avoid vaccinating animals. This behavior needs to change in order to control and minimize the recurrent impact of the disease in these countries.

Immunization after vaccination is likely to persist for two, 3 years but since effective experimental demonstrations are still missing, manufacturers recommended vaccinating animals annually.[50]

Antibody responses resulting from LSDV vaccines and wild-type LSDV are, to date, indistinguishable by serology (DIVA "differentiating infected from vaccinated animals" testing), which can be problematic. Vaccinated animals are subject to movement restrictions by national trade legislation, thus resulting in economic losses for farmers and stakeholders.

Empirical experience in the field demonstrated that mass vaccination with homologous vaccines seems to be the most effective control policy when applied in concert with other control measures, such as limits of movement and depopulation strategies.[22]

Animal Movement Restrictions

Movement of mild, asymptomatic infected animals is an important route of spread for LSDV from an infected area to a free one. Uncontrolled movement of animals represents one of the major risks of spreading LSD in free territories. Pastoralism, nomadic movement, and illegal trade of animals should be assessed.

Animals moving to territories with a higher health status should always be tested for LSD and are subject to veterinary inspection and completion of an appropriate health certificate. Full immunization is achieved 28 days after vaccination, so animals should not be moved until that time. On the other hand, certain animals cannot be fully protected after vaccination, for different reasons such as pathologic or physiologic conditions, or problems in handling and administration of the vaccine. For these reasons, vaccinated animals should be tested and are free from LSD before allowing transportation to territories with a higher health status.

In the European Union, in case of outbreaks, the movement of animals is completely banned (with the appropriate exceptions) into the perimeter of protection and surveillance zones of 20 and 50 km radius, respectively, as established by European Regulation.[51]

In free countries, surveillance on animals moved from other countries is the most important measure of control against LSD.

Depopulation Strategies

Depopulation of animals is a widely used control measure, with differing results dependent on the circumstances of the campaign in which it is applied. Culling animals can reduce virus circulation, but because of the vector-borne nature of the disease, it will not stop virus circulation indefinitely. For this reason, it should never be the only measure used.

Total stamping out was applied during the Balkans epidemic before the vaccination campaign began. After initiating vaccination, if it is properly applied, total or partial stamping out does not show differences in the resolution of the outbreaks, as also demonstrated by mathematical models.[29] Stamping out must be evaluated with particular attention because of its huge economic, moral, and environmental impact.

Because animals showing symptoms are considered the main source of virus for hematophagous insects, the strategy of partial stamping out has been adopted, especially during vaccination campaigns. Laboratory confirmation to distinguish infected animals with wild strain from vaccinates is preferred, together with a humane culling procedure and proper disposal of carcasses. Nevertheless, the identification of sick animals can be difficult when symptoms and signs are mild, but the transmission capacity of these individuals is uncertain.

As assessed by the European Food Safety Authority in 2021, preventive culling of animals should be applied to reduce the likelihood of undetected spread in three cases *(1) in an establishment where LSD is suspected, (2) in the establishments in temporary restricted zones, and (3) in the establishments of the restricted zones (ie, the protection and surveillance zones and further restricted zones).*[29]

Biosecurity Measures

Proper cleaning and disinfection during outbreaks are important activities for outbreak resolution in order to avoid the recurrence of the infection. Even if the disease is vector-mediated, biosecurity measures can still reduce the risk of a new outbreak.

LSDV contained in nodules is scattered in the environment where it can persist for long periods, especially in stables and barns where animals are kept.[52] In necrotic nodules, LSDV persists for up to 33 days or longer, in desiccated crust for up to 35 days and at least 18 days in air-dried hides. The virus is susceptible to sunlight and detergents containing lipid solvents.[3] The control of the vectors is difficult because of the great number of different species involved in the transmission, some of which are still unknown. Otherwise, regular manners applied inside the facilities and in the surrounding areas can help to minimize the densities of insects that come in close contact with animals. Removing and avoiding the insects' breeding sites such as stagnant water, manure piles, and slurry, using mosquito trapping and netting at the windows, and applying of insecticides on cattle are all possible strategies to control the number of vectors in the herd.[53]

Treatment

Treatment of symptomatic animals is possible, in order to save lives but not always effective in reducing the spread of the disease in the farms as well as in the regions. Mildly sick animals should recover spontaneously without any treatment. Severely sick animals need good quality feed and care whenever this is possible. Antibiotics can be administered in order to prevent secondary bacterial infections. Treatment of sick animals is applicable when the number of sick animals is very low or in the case of a valuable animal. Cattle with severe forms of disease have low chances of recovery, so treatment may not be advisable in these animals.

CLINICS CARE POINTS

- Clinical symptoms that appear after the incubation period can be grouped into 4 phases. In the first acute phase, which occurs for 7 to 10 days, symptoms are high fever (41°C), anorexia, lacrimation, depression, increased nasal discharge, decreased milk, increased saliva secretion, and multinodular lesions found around the skin and mucous membranes. In the second phase, swelling of the subscapular and precrural lymph nodes occurs, as well as an increase in the number of nodules. In the third phase, 2 to 3 weeks from the beginning of symptoms, nodules ulcerate and necrose. In the fourth phase, after at least 1 month, ulceration, skin thickening, and hyperpigmentation of the lesions occur.

- The samples used to detect lumpy skin disease virus DNA by polymerase chain reaction (PCR) or RT-PCR methods are skin nodules, secretions, and blood from infected animals. Following the first appearance of the skin lesions, the virus can be isolated for up to 35 days and viral nucleic acid can be demonstrated via PCR for up to 3 months.

- Vaccination and control of animal movement are the most important control measures to stop the spread of the disease and to avoid its entrance into free territories.

- No treatment is available for the virus. Where deemed appropriate, sick animals can be treated with antibiotics to reduce the risk of secondary infections and fluids administered to support the metabolic recovery.

ACKNOWLEDGMENTS

The authors would like to thank Dr Massimo Scacchia, Head of the Cooperation, Research and Development Unit and expert at WOAH Reference Laboratory for Bovine Contagious bovine pleuropneumonia (CBPP) at Istituto Zooprofilattico Sperimentale dell'Abruzzo e del Molise "Giuseppe Caporale" (IZSAM) for the beautiful pictures collected during his huge field experience in African countries. The authors would also thank Dr Daniela Morelli, Head of National Reference Center for the study and verification of Foreign Animal Diseases (CESME) and Dr Federica Monaco, Head of Diagnosis and surveillance of viral diseases Unit of IZSAM for sharing their experience in the diagnosis of the disease.

DISCLOSURE

The authors have nothing to disclose.

REFERENCES

1. Mulatu E, Feyisa A. Review: Lumpy skin disease. J Vet Sci Technol 2018; 9(535):1–8.
2. World Organisation for Animal Health, (WOAH). Lumpy skin disease technical card. Last updated June 2022.
3. World organization for animal health (WOAH). Manual of Diagnostic Tests and Vaccines for Terrestrial Animals. Chapter 3.4.12: Lumpy Skin Disease. Last update 2023.
4. National animal health reporting system (NAHRS) by the United States Animal Health Association, American Association of Veterinary Laboratory Diagnosticians, and Animal and Plant National Inspection Service.Voluntary 2023 U.S. reportable diseases, infections, and infestations list.
5. HHS (United States Deprtment of Health and Human Services) and USDA (United States Department of Agricolture) select agents and toxins 7 CFR part 331, 9 CFR part 121, and 42 CFR part 73. Last Reviewed: August 1, 2023.
6. Bianchini J, Simons X, Humblet M, et al. Lumpy skin disease: A systematic review of mode of transmission, risk of emergence and risk entry pathway. Viruses 2023; 15(8):1622.
7. El-Nahas E, El-Habbaa A, El-Bagoury G, et al. Isolation and identification of lumpy skin disease virus from naturally infected buffaloes at Kaluobia, Egypt. Global Vet 2011;7:234–7.
8. Carn VM, Kitching RP. An investigation of possible routes of transmission of lumpy skin disease virus (Neethling). Epidemiol Infect 1995;114(1):219–26.
9. Barnard BJ. Antibodies against some viruses of domestic animals in southern African wild animals. Onderstepoort J Vet Res 1997;64(2):95–110.
10. Duvallet G, Hogsette JA. Global diversity, distribution, and genetic studies of stable flies (stomoxys sp.). Diversity 2023;15(5):600.
11. Laporta GZ, Potter AM, Oliveira JFA, et al. Global distribution of aedes aegypti and aedes albopictus in a climate change scenario of regional rivalry. Insects 2023;14(1):49.

12. Chihota CM, Rennie LF, Kitching RP, et al. Attempted mechanical transmission of lumpy skin disease virus by biting insects. Med Vet Entomol 2003;17(3): 294–300.
13. Sanz-Bernardo B, Haga IR, Wijesiriwardana N, et al. Quantifying and modeling the acquisition and retention of lumpy skin disease virus by hematophagus insects reveals clinically but not subclinically affected cattle are promoters of viral transmission and key targets for control of disease outbreaks. J Virol 2021;95(9): e022399-e2320.
14. Sanz-Bernardo B, Suckoo R, Haga IR, et al. The acquisition and retention of lumpy skin disease virus by blood-feeding insects is influenced by the source of virus, the insect body part, and the time since feeding. J Virol 2022;96(15): e0075122-22.
15. Service M. Medical entomology for students, 2008, Cambridge University Press, 111–120.
16. Magori-Cohen R, Louzoun Y, Herziger Y, et al. Mathematical modelling and evaluation of the different routes of transmission of lumpy skin disease virus. Vet Res 2012;43(1):1.
17. Rouby S, Aboulsoud E. Evidence of intrauterine transmission of lumpy skin disease virus. Vet J 2016;209:193–5.
18. Gari G, Waret-Szkuta A, Grosbois V, et al. Risk factors associated with observed clinical lumpy skin disease in Ethiopia. Epidemiol Infect 2010;138(11):1657–66.
19. Ma J, Yuan Y, Shao J, et al. Genomic characterization of lumpy skin disease virus in southern china. Transbound Emerg Dis 2022;69(5):2788–99.
20. Tuppurainen E, Alexandrov T, Beltrán-Alcrudo D. A manual for veterinarians. FAO animal production and health manual no. 20. rome: food and agriculture organization of the united nations (FAO); 2017.
21. Food E, Authority S, Calistri P, et al. Lumpy skin disease II. data collection and analysis. EFSA J 2018;16(2):e05176.
22. European Food Safety Authority, (EFSA), Calistri P, De Clercq K, Gubbins S, et al. Lumpy skin disease epidemiological report IV: Data collection and analysis. EFSA J 2020;18(2):e06010.
23. Coetzer JAW, Tustin RC. Infectious diseases of livestock. 2nd edition. Cape Town (South Africa): Oxford University Press Cape Town; 2004. https://worldcat.org/title/57541742.
24. Yeruham I, Nir O, Braverman Y, et al. Spread of lumpy skin disease in Israeli dairy herds. Vet Rec 1995;137(4):91–3.
25. World Animal Health Information System(WAHIS), Available online at https://wahis.woah.org/#/home Updated in 2023.
26. Kumar N, Chander Y, Kumar R, et al. Isolation and characterization of lumpy skin disease virus from cattle in India. PLoS One 2021;16(1):e0241022.
27. Şevik M, Doğan M. Epidemiological and molecular studies on lumpy skin disease outbreaks in turkey during 2014-2015. Transbound Emerg Dis 2017;64(4): 1268–79.
28. Sukoco H, Fahrodi DU, Said NS, et al. Lumpy skin disease (LSD): Etiology, pathogenesis, prevention and control. JETISH 2023;2(1):549–60.
29. European Food Safety Authority. EFSA panel assessment of the control measures for category A diseases of animal health law lumpy skin 2022.
30. Liang Z, Yao K, Wang S, et al. Understanding the research advances on lumpy skin disease: A comprehensive literature review of experimental evidence. Front Microbiol 2022;13:1065894.

31. Babiuk S, Bowden TR, Parkyn G, et al. Quantification of lumpy skin disease virus following experimental infection in cattle. Transbound Emerg Dis 2008;55(7): 299–307.

32. Khalafalla A. Lumpy skin disease: An economically significant emerging disease. Veterinary Medicine and Science 2023. https://doi.org/10.5772/intechopen. 108845.

33. Tuppurainen ESM, Venter EH, Shisler JL, et al. Review: Capripoxvirus diseases: Current status and opportunities for control. Transbound Emerg Dis 2017;64(3): 729–45.

34. Ahmed AM, Dessoukki AA. Dessouki. Abattoir-based survey and histopatholog-ical findings of lumpy skin disease in cattle at Ismailia Abattoir. Int J Biosci Bio-chem Bioinforma 2013;3(4):372.

35. Abutarbush SM, Ababneh MM, Al Zoubi IG, et al. Lumpy skin disease in Jordan: Disease emergence, clinical signs, complications and preliminary-associated economic losses. Transbound Emerg Dis 2015;62(5):549–54.

36. Jalali SM, Rasooli A, Seifi Abad Shapuri M, et al. Clinical, hematologic, and biochemical findings in cattle infected with lumpy skin disease during an outbreak in southwest Iran. Arch Razi Inst 2017;72(4):255–65.

37. Gaber A, Rouby S, Elsaied A, et al. Assessment of heterologous lumpy skin dis-ease vaccine-induced immunity in pregnant cattle vaccinated at different times of gestation period and their influence on maternally derived antibodies. Vet Immu-nol Immunopathol 2022;244:110380.

38. Tuppurainen ESM, Venter EH, Coetzer JAW. The detection of lumpy skin disease virus in samples of experimentally infected cattle using different diagnostic tech-niques. Onderstepoort J Vet Res 2005;72(2):153–64.

39. Agianniotaki EI, Babiuk S, Katsoulos PD, et al. Panagiotis-Dimitrios Katsoulos, Colostrum transfer of neutralizing antibodies against lumpy skin disease virus from vaccinated cows to their calves. Transboundary and Emerging Diseases 2018;65(6):2043–8.

40. Moudgil G, Chadha J, Khullar L, et al. Lumpy skin disease: Insights into current status and geographical expansion of a transboundary viral disease, Microbial Pathogenesis, 106485, 2023.

41. Flannery J, Shih B, Haga IR, et al. A novel strain of lumpy skin disease virus causes clinical disease in cattle in Hong Kong. Transbound Emerg Dis 2022; 69(4):e336–43.

42. Van Schalkwyk A, Byadovskaya O, Shumilova I, et al. Estimating evolutionary changes between highly passaged and original parental lumpy skin disease virus strains. Transbound Emerg Dis 2022;69(4):e486–96.

43. van Schalkwyk A, Kara P, Ebersohn K, et al. Potential link of single nucleotide polymorphisms to virulence of vaccine-associated field strains of lumpy skin dis-ease virus in South Africa. Transbound Emerg Dis 2020;67(6):2946–60.

44. Ben-Gera J, Klement E, Khinich E, et al. Comparison of the efficacy of Neethling lumpy skin disease virus and x10RM65 sheep-pox live attenuated vaccines for the prevention of lumpy skin disease - the results of a randomized controlled field study. Vaccine 2015;33(38):4837–42.

45. WEISS KE. Lumpy skin disease virus. Virology Monographs, 1968;3:111–131.

46. Katsoulos P, Chaintoutis SC, Dovas CI, et al. Investigation on the incidence of adverse reactions, viraemia and haematological changes following field immuni-zation of cattle using a live attenuated vaccine against lumpy skin disease. Trans-bound Emerg Dis 2018;65(1):174–85.

47. Tasioudi KE, Antoniou SE, Iliadou P, et al. Emergence of lumpy skin disease in greece 2015. Transbound Emerg Dis 2016;63(3):260–5.
48. Food E, Authority S, Stegeman JA, et al. Lumpy skin disease I. data collection and analysis. EFSA J 2018;16(2):e05176.
49. Regulation (EU) 2016/429 of the European parliament and of the council of 9 march 2016 on transmissible animal diseases and amending and repealing certain acts in the area of animal health ('Animal health law').
50. Tuppurainen E, Dietze K, Wolff J, et al. Review: Vaccines and vaccination against lumpy skin disease. Vaccines (Basel) 2021;9(10):1136.
51. Delegated regulation 2020/687 of 17 December 2019 supplementing regulation (EU) 2016/429 of the European parliament and the council, as regards rules for the prevention and control of certain listed diseases.
52. JAW Coetzer and P Oberem (Directors) In: Infectious Diseases of Livestock, JAW Coetzer, GR Thomson,NJ Maclachlan and M-L Penrith (Editors).JAW Coetzer, E Tupparainen, S Babiuk, D B WALLACE. Lumpy skin disease. 2018.Anipedia, www.anipedia.org.
53. FAO (Food and Agricoltural Organization of the United Nations), Sustainable prevention, control and elimination of Lumpy Skin Disease - Eastern Europe and the Balkans. FAO Animal Production and Health Position Paper. No, 2, 2017.

Contagious Bovine Pleuropneumonia

Global Eradication Remains a Challenging and Distant Goal

Ahmed El Idrissi Hamzi, DVM, PhD[a],*, Akiko Kamata, DVM, MSc[b],
William Amanfu, DVM, MSc[c]

KEYWORDS

- Contagious bovine pleuropneumonia • CBPP • Control • Eradication
- Epidemiology

KEY POINTS

- Contagious bovine pleuropneumonia (CBPP) is eradicated in most continents including North America.
- Africa is currently the only continent where CBPP is prevalent, within areas south of the Sahara and north of the South African region.
- Control or elimination of the disease can be achieved by various strategies including vaccination, movement control, and stamping-out.
- Although CBPP has been successfully eliminated from Europe, North America, and Australia using a combination of strictly enforced movement controls and test and slaughter, these approaches are difficult to implement in the context of the African countries where the disease is endemic.
- National governments, private stakeholders, regional bodies, international intergovernmental organizations, and funding partners are encouraged to invest in CBPP control as a basis for improving food security and people's livelihoods, and therefore contributing to achieving Sustainable Development Goals.

INTRODUCTION

Contagious bovine pleuropneumonia (CBPP), also known as lung sickness, is an infectious and contagious respiratory disease of cattle caused by *Mycoplasma mycoides* subsp. *mycoides* (Mmm). With the eradication of rinderpest in 2011, CBPP has become

[a] International Animal Health Expert, Rome, Italy; [b] The Food and Agriculture Organization of the United Nations, Viale delle Terme di Caracalla 00153, Rome, Italy; [c] International Veterinary Consultant, Accra, Ghana
* Corresponding author.
E-mail address: elidrissi702@gmail.com

Vet Clin Food Anim 40 (2024) 277–291
https://doi.org/10.1016/j.cvfa.2024.01.003
0749-0720/24/© 2024 Elsevier Inc. All rights reserved.
vetfood.theclinics.com

the most serious threat to cattle production in sub-Saharan Africa where the disease remains endemic. CBPP has been eradicated from most continents. The United States eliminated CBPP in 1892 after an intensive quarantine and slaughter program.[1]

CBPP is a disease with very high economic importance, with severe implications for food security and livelihoods in endemic areas. The impact of CBPP on farmers and the economy is significant, costing millions of dollars annually in Africa due to direct and indirect production losses attributed to morbidity and mortality plus the disease control cost.[2]

The disease is transmitted by direct or close contact between infected cattle and susceptible animals. Clinically, the disease is characterized by an acute or subacute pleuropneumonia with considerable variations in severity of signs observed in affected animals. Surviving cattle often become carriers that can form potential sources for introduction of the pathogen into uninfected herds.[3]

Control or elimination of the disease can be achieved by various strategies including vaccination, movement control, and stamping-out. These approaches are underpinned by surveillance, availability of diagnostics, and animal identification. In many sub-Saharan African countries where the disease is endemic, control of CBPP has been constrained by several factors including the deterioration in the quality of veterinary services, lack of financial resources to mount sustained control programs, and uncontrolled cattle movement within and between countries. As a result, many countries in sub-Saharan Africa are still struggling with this disease, compromising continental and global eradication.[4,5] The disease is a barrier to regional and international trade of live animals in many countries in Africa.

In this review, basic epidemiologic features and clinical signs of CBPP are presented and disease control challenges are briefly discussed.

GEOGRAPHIC DISTRIBUTION

The first reported case of CBPP was in 1693 in Germany. The disease then spread from Germany to all over Europe, and subsequently to North America, Africa, Australia in the mid-nineteenth century and then to Asia in the early twentieth century through colonial activities and trade.[6] CBPP entered the United States in 1843 and by 1884, the disease was so widespread that the federal government established the Bureau of Animal Industry (which later developed into the United States Department of Agriculture's [USDA] Animal and Plant Health Inspection Service [APHIS]) to eliminate the disease from the country.[7] The first intensive campaign to control an animal disease by quarantine and slaughter began in 1887 with CBPP, and the disease was successfully eradicated from the United States in 1892.

After elimination of the disease from Europe in the nineteenth century, the disease reappeared in Portugal and Spain in 1951 and 1957, respectively. A few outbreaks were reported in France, with the latest in 1984. In Italy, the disease reappeared in 1990 but was eliminated by 1993, and the last case in Europe was in Portugal in 1999.[6]

CBPP has also been reported in several countries of the Middle East and the Arabian Peninsula, probably caused by cattle imported from some countries in Africa. CBPP was also reported by a few countries in Asia, namely India, Bangladesh, Myanmar, Nepal, and China.[3] The situation in Eastern Europe is unclear although many countries have indicated they are, or officially declared (eg, the Russian Federation), free of CBPP.

Today, CBPP is present in Central, East, West, and parts of Southern Africa. According to the World Organisation for Animal Health (WOAH) reports, there are currently about 25 sub-Saharan African countries with cases of CBPP. In Africa, CBPP is found in an area south of the Sahara Desert from the Tropic of Cancer in the north to the Tropic of Capricorn in the south.[5] Due to the lack of rigorous surveillance and control programs, CBPP is now emerging in disease-free areas and its incidence is increasing within endemic zones. Countries that have reported CBPP from 2019 to 2023 and those implementing vaccination are shown in **Fig. 1**.

EPIDEMIOLOGY AND IMPACT OF CONTAGIOUS BOVINE PLEUROPNEUMONIA
Pathogen

CBPP is caused by *Mycoplasma mycoides* subsp. *mycoides* (Mmm), which belongs to the *Mycoplasma mycoides* cluster. This cluster consists of 5 mycoplasma species or subspecies from bovines, sheep, and goats that share serologic and genetic characteristics. Like all mycoplasmas, Mmm lacks a cell wall and is therefore pleomorphic and resistant to antibiotics of the beta-lactam group, such as penicillin. Culture of mycoplasma is quite slow (several days) and requires special growth media.[8] Selective culture media, supplemented with penicillin G and thallium acetate, can be used to isolate Mmm from contaminated samples.[9] Mmm is easily inactivated by most common disinfectants for example, by mercuric chloride (0.01%/1 min), phenol (1%/3 min), and formaldehyde solution (0.5%/30 s). Survival of Mmm in the environment depends on the climate; it survives for a short time (up to 3 days) in tropical areas and up to 2 weeks in temperate zones.[8]

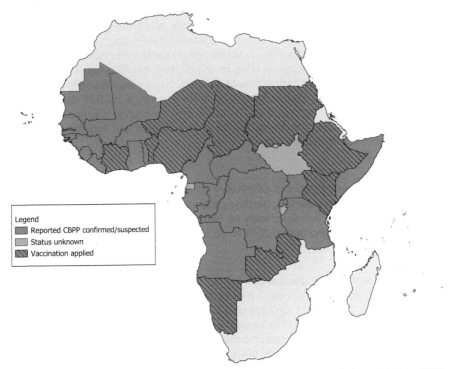

Fig. 1. Countries that have reported the disease during the period from 2019 to 2023. (World Organisation for Animal Health (WOAH) (2023). - WAHIS Official Disease Status. Retrieved from https://www.woah.org/en/what-we-do/animal-health-and-welfare/official-disease-status/. Screenshot or copy by Elsevier. Reproduced with permission. The World Organisation for Animal Health (WOAH) bears no responsibility for the integrity or accuracy of the data contained herein, but not limited to, any deletion, manipulation, or reformatting of data that may have occurred beyond its control.)

Host Species and Susceptibility

Cattle—bovine (*Bos taurus*) or zebu (*Bos indicus*)—domestic buffalo (*Bubalus bubalis*), captive bison (*Bison bison*), and yak are all susceptible to CBPP, but only cattle play an important role in the epidemiology of the disease.[9] Wild bovids, in particular the African water buffalo (*Syncerus caffer*), are resistant to CBPP and no wild animals have ever been involved in the epidemiologic cycle.[8] Small ruminants are potential reservoirs of the pathogen, although transmission of CBPP from these species to cattle has never been reported.[3] Humans are not susceptible to CBPP infection.

Introduction and Transmission

The disease appears in a herd either after the introduction of an infected animal or after cattle have been herded together at water holes or common grazing areas. Once introduced, CBPP may evolve undetected for several months. Due to individual variations in susceptibility and to the long incubation period (2 weeks to 4 months), the evolution of CBPP within a herd is irregular and insidious, with latent carriers often maintaining the disease.

The sources of the pathogen are diseased domestic animals or latent carriers with sequestra. Contamination requires close contact between excreting and susceptible animals. Transmission of CBPP is mainly by aerosol through nasal discharge and bronchial secretions when animals cough. Indirect transmission by infected premises, contaminated pastures, fodder, water, animal waste, and fomites plays a minor role, if any, in the spread of the disease.[3] Distant contamination through airborne spread up to 200 m is thought to be possible. Transplacental infection has been known to occur and the agent can be detected in urine or semen, fetal membranes, and uterine discharges; however, the real importance of these routes of transmission in the epidemiology of the disease is negligible.[9] The role of climate change in CBPP disease spread and control has not yet been studied. However, climate change is expected to impact animal movements and thus disease spread since drought and flooding are essential determinants of cattle movements.[4,10]

Prevalence

The prevalence and incidence of CBPP vary according to the cattle production system factors including cattle density, herding patterns, and environmental conditions.[7] In areas where CBPP is endemic such as different sub-Saharan African countries.,[11] prevalence rates ranging from 0.29% to 10.5% have been reported.

Impact

In affected countries, the disease has serious implications for food security and livelihoods caused by mortality, loss of milk production, and drastic weight loss in more chronic cases. The impact on agricultural production and consequential reduced food supply is also the result of reduced draught power.[12] CBPP is a barrier to regional and international trade which reduces the value of livestock and the income of many stakeholders along the livestock value chain. The disease has significant socioeconomic impacts on demand and supply, food security, and nutrition. The presence of CBPP also poses a constant threat to CBPP-free countries and generates costs incurred to the implementation of sanitary measures necessary to control and eliminate the disease.[13]

The economic impact of CBPP has been estimated by Tambi and colleagues[2] in 12 sub-Saharan countries that reported the vast majority of CBPP outbreaks. Results of this study showed significant impact on farmers and the economy due to direct and indirect production losses plus the disease control costs. The total annual economic cost of CBPP in these countries has been estimated to be about 45 million US dollars.

Despite these studies, accurate evaluation of the losses due to CBPP in endemic countries is difficult because of the lack of proper and consistent disease reporting and specific data, especially at the national level, on the impact of the disease. The cost/benefit analysis of control programs are lacking. Evaluation of the real epidemiologic situation and economic losses of CBPP at the herd and community levels is a critical step for developing an effective control program for CBPP. Broad-based impact assessment studies of CBPP are needed for better decision-making regarding CBPP control at national and international levels.[7]

CLINICAL SIGNS AND EVOLUTION OF THE DISEASE
Clinical Forms of Contagious Bovine Pleuropneumonia

Clinical signs vary depending on the pathogenicity of the mycoplasma strain and the susceptibility of the animals (breed, age, and immune status). There is considerable variation in severity of signs observed in cattle affected by CBPP, ranging from peracute through acute to subacute, chronic, and sub-clinical forms. Peracute CBPP is rare and cattle may die within a week due to the abundant pleural and pericardial effusion, with no significant clinical signs other than fever.[9] The acute form commonly occurs at the beginning of an epidemic where the animal shows anorexia, a fall in milk production, irregular rumination, fever, and difficulty breathing. As the disease progresses, the signs become more pronounced with increased respiratory rate, short breaths, painful coughing, and grunting at expiration. These signs are exacerbated when the animal is forced to rise or to move. The animal becomes prostrate or stands with the back arched, head extended, and elbows turned out (**Fig. 2**). After 1 to 3 weeks, the animal may die or enter a chronic phase. In calves, pulmonary localization is rare, and animals may present primarily with polyarthritis that is evident as swelling of carpal and hock joints and lameness ensues.[3]

In some cases, clinical signs are less severe and less specific and may be limited to a slight temporary rise in body temperature, loss of condition, and a mild cough noticeable when the animal is exercised. CBPP may evolve to a chronic state with regression of the clinical signs and encapsulation of the pulmonary lesions with possible full recovery after several weeks and even months. Cattle recovering from CBPP can play a role in disease spread within the herd.[3]

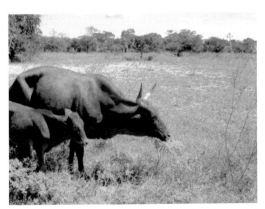

Fig. 2. Clinical CBPP (Extended neck and abducted forelimbs of the adult cow). (Source: William Amanfu.)

Morbidity and Mortality

CBPP morbidity rates vary between herds depending on the epidemiologic situation and the severity of the disease. In endemic areas, morbidity rates are often low (below 10%), whereas during an epidemic outbreak, morbidity rates can be much higher in naïve populations. Death is not usually the outcome of the disease, but high mortality rates of up to 90% may be observed in the peracute form of the disease. In the acute and subclinical forms, the mortality rates are usually lower.[14]

Post Mortem Findings

The principal post mortem lesions of CBPP include inflammation of the pleura (pleuritis) and thickening and inflammation of lung tissues. Large amounts of straw-colored fluid mixed with fibrin flakes may be present in the thoracic cavity and the lung, and the parietal pleura is often covered by thick deposits of fibrin. On cross-section of the lung, the typical marbled appearance is evident because of the widened interlobular septa. In the chronic form, sequestra (2–30 cm in diameter) are composed of necrotic lung tissue surrounded by a fibrous capsule (**Fig. 3**). Gross pathologic lesions of the lung are typical and often unilateral.[8] In young animals, the principal lesion is polyarthritis with synovitis.[3]

DIAGNOSIS

Diagnosis of CBPP is based on the epidemiologic context of the disease, clinical signs, post-mortem findings, and laboratory confirmation. While the peracute and acute forms of the disease are relatively easy to recognize, diagnosis can be challenging in areas where the disease is endemic and most often is subclinical or chronic. Pathologic findings are of great value for a rapid presumptive diagnosis but laboratory analyses are always essential to confirm or to rule out CBPP, especially when it is suspected in disease-free areas. The simultaneous presence of pulmonary symptoms in adults and polyarthritis in calves should be considered highly suggestive of the disease.[8] CBPP frequently results in disease in only 1 lung as compared with other types of pneumonia in which both lungs are affected. It is necessary to differentiate the disease from other diseases that may present similar clinical signs or lesions. Primary differential diagnoses are summarized in **Table 1**.[3,15]

Confirmatory diagnosis is based on the isolation of Mmm from clinical samples of the lung. Mmm can be isolated from nasal swabs or discharge of live animals. At

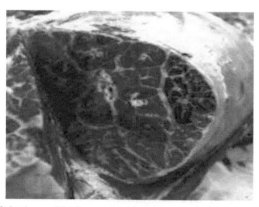

Fig. 3. Marbling of the lungs (Thickened interlobular space). (Source William Amanfu.)

Table 1
Differential diagnoses for CBPP[3,15]

Disease	Clinical Signs and Lesions that May be Confused with CBPP		
	Clinical Signs	Lesions	Element of Differentiation
Rinderpest	• Fever and discharges observed from the eyes, nose, and mouth	• Red areas of lung collapse together with emphysema of lobules and the septa separating them	• Rinderpest globally eradicated • Erosions in the mouth and throughout the digestive tract, together with the profuse, often bloody diarrhea in advanced cases of rinderpest are not seen in CBPP
Bovine pneumonic pasteurellosis (Mannheimia hemolytic and Pasteurella multocida) or Hemorrhagic septicemia (Pasteurella multocida)	• Fever Hypersalivation Nasal discharge • Labored respiration, Depression, and weakness	• Serofibrinous pleural exudate and fibrinous to fibrinopurulent bronchopneumonia • Widespread congestion with petechiae and ecchymoses in tissues and on serosal surfaces • Sequestrum formation in chronic forms can appear very similar to the marbling lesion of CBPP	• Pasteurellosis most commonly affects young animals • Pasteurellosis is an acute disease and generally spreads more rapidly through a herd than CBPP. • Edema of the throat and neck to the brisket is often very pronounced and not seen in CBPP • The pneumonic lesions are often bilateral (unlike CBPP) • In pasteurellosis, stained impression smears of affected lung tissue reveal the typical bipolar rod-like bacteria, which will usually be isolated in pure culture on standard blood agar medium
Theileriosis (East Coast fever, ECF)	• Clinical signs of respiratory distress Fever • Coughing, • Nasal and ocular discharge • Diarrhea	• Lung edema • General enlargement of superficial lymph nodes and especially those of the head	• In ECF, there is a severe lung edema with much clear liquid, which is also present in the chest cavity • Neither pneumonia nor inflammation of the pleura is present

(continued on next page)

Table 1
(continued)

Disease	Clinical Signs	Lesions	Element of Differentiation
		Clinical Signs and Lesions that May be Confused with CBPP	
Bovine malignant catarrhal fever (MCF)	• Fever • Oral and nasal erosions • Enlarged lymph nodes • Corneal opacity	• Inflammation and necrosis of respiratory, alimentary, or urinary mucosal epithelium • Generalized lymphoid proliferation and necrosis	• MCF is a disease of domestic cattle, water buffalo, American bison, and deer • A patchy pneumonia may be seen in cases of MCF
Ephemeral fever (EF)	• Fever • Serous discharges from the nose and eyes • Salivation • Lameness and swollen joints • Pulmonary emphysema	• Polyserositis affecting pleural, pericardial, and peritoneal surfaces • Serofibrinous polysynovitis and polyarthritis	• In most cases EF is a self-limiting disease of short duration • Noncontagious, disease affecting cattle and water buffalo • Pneumonia is not a main feature of the disease but secondary pneumonia can occur with lung edema and emphysema in some cases • Swollen joints can occur in animals of all ages, unlike CBPP
Tuberculosis	• Emaciation (cachexia) • Anorexia • Irregular breathing in chronic cases with frequent coughing	• Tubercular nodules are degenerative cheese-like lesions, sometimes calcified	• The capsule of the tubercular nodules is not well defined when compared to that of CBPP sequestra
Echinococcosis		• Old, thickly encapsulated hydatid cysts	• Echinococcal cysts have a double wall and contain a clear liquid, often calcified when old

necropsy, pleural fluid is the sample of choice followed by bronchial mucus, diseased lung, and lymph nodes draining the respiratory tract. Samples can be frozen or immediately transported to the laboratory in cold boxes at +4°C (39.2°F). Isolation of Mmm can be performed by inoculating appropriate media with pleural fluid or ground-up lung lesions. Identification of Mmm can be done by conventional biochemical and immunologic tests or increasingly by polymerase chain reaction (PCR) assay. Serologic diagnosis can be performed by different techniques including complement fixation test (CFT), competitive enzyme-linked immunosorbent assay (c-ELISA), and slide agglutination test.[8] Training that empowers disease recognition, data collection, as well as reporting through increased awareness is an essential pre-requisite to effective sustainable diagnostic capability for CBPP.

CONTAGIOUS BOVINE PLEUROPNEUMONIA CONTROL AND ELIMINATION
Disease Reporting

CBPP is a disease listed by WOAH in the Terrestrial Animal Health Code (Terrestrial Code). Members are obligated to report occurrences of the disease according to the standards and procedures in the Terrestrial Code.

CBPP is a notifiable disease in many countries around the world, and veterinarians who encounter or suspect the disease should follow their national guidelines for disease reporting. In the United States, state or federal veterinary authorities should be informed immediately when there is a suspicion of the disease.[1]

Elimination and Control Programs

In countries free from CBPP, the only control measure is the strict prohibition of the import of animals from infected countries or areas. While this measure is easy to enforce in some countries, it may be difficult to implement in countries where nomadism and cross-border animal movements are practiced in transhumance cattle production systems. When the disease is introduced in a country, severe control measures are necessary, such as quarantine and culling of all infected herds and exposed animals. Effective implementation of these measures has allowed elimination/eradication of CBPP in many countries such as the United States, United Kingdom, and Western Europe without the aid of diagnostic tests (for detection of infected animals) and vaccination. Elimination of the disease in these countries required intense commitment combined with rigorous enforcement of movement control and stamping out procedures (**Table 2**).

Other measures that have been applied to control and eliminate the disease include various combinations of identification and slaughter of infected animals, vaccination, and movement control. This approach was used over several years in Australia where massive vaccination campaigns significantly reduced the prevalence of the disease before shifting to implementation of a strict stamping out policy that led to the elimination of the disease from the country.[16] Similar models based on identification and slaughter of infected animals were employed in South Africa where herds were isolated in the field and animals were tested by the CFT. Positive animals were immediately slaughtered.[7] Similarly, in Botswana, clinical and abattoir surveillance combined with strictly enforced stamping out measures enabled the elimination of CBPP from the country after its reappearance in 1995.[17]

In most sub-Saharan African countries where CBPP is endemic, strictly enforced movement control and culling are not easily applicable due to the specific socioeconomic conditions. Vaccination is the only method to limit the spread of disease and reduce the prevalence to a level low enough to enable implementation of radical

Table 2
Eradication schemes in selected countries

Country	Date of Eradication/ Elimination	Eradication Strategy
USA	1892	Clinical identification, intensive quarantine, elimination of suspect cases, and disinfection of premises
United Kingdom	1898	Movement control and slaughter of infected and in-contact cattle
Australia	1968	Vaccination followed by strict test and slaughter
China	1989	Vaccination with attenuated vaccine
Western Europe	Beginning of twentieth Century. No report since the last case in Portugal in 1999	Abattoir surveillance, movement control, and slaughter of infected and contact animals
South Africa	1924	Detection of infected animals and slaughter of positive cases
Botswana	1939 (reappeared in 1995) and eliminated in 1998	Clinical and abattoir surveillance. Stamping out measures

elimination procedures. The commercial vaccines available are live and attenuated T1/44 and T1/SR vaccine strains. The former is more widely used, as it provides protection for a year, while the duration of immunity of the T1/SR vaccine is shorter. The T1/44 vaccine may sometimes induce a postvaccine local reaction, particularly in animals vaccinated for the first time. The latter (T1/SR) has the advantage of inducing fewer adverse local reactions but requires revaccinations to induce strong protection. The protective immunity of both vaccines is cell mediated, and antibody response is short-lived and limited.[18,19] Despite their limitations, these vaccines can provide sufficient protection if properly deployed by using the correct dosage and ensuring efficient delivery of the vaccines under appropriate cold chain maintenance protocols.[12]

Surveillance is essential for formulating a strategy, detecting events, defining epidemiologic zones within a country, and measuring progress. Surveillance methods include abattoir surveillance, sero-surveillance with the competitive ELISA or CFT, and participatory surveillance.[12] Abattoir surveillance, particularly in at-risk areas, can serve as a powerful surveillance tool to detect CBPP cases and estimate the prevalence based on post mortem findings. Promoting syndromic surveillance at abattoirs/slaughter facilities at the field level (district, region) is essential in countries with limited resources.

Treatment

The inability to control the disease using vaccines alone in certain areas has precipitated discussions to assess the effectiveness of the use of antibiotics in the management of CBPP outbreaks.[12,20,21] The use of antibiotics was discouraged long ago based on the perception that antibiotic treatment may predispose infected cattle to develop sequestra in their lung or may cause infected animals to become chronic carriers, therefore creating potential sources of infection and spread of the disease. In addition, antibiotics used to treat other diseases may impact the expression of CBPP in animals. Despite the official condemnation in using antibiotics to treat CBPP, there is evidence of widespread antibiotic treatment by farmers in the field to treat CBPP.[22] Several studies have been conducted on the use of antibiotics for the treatment of the disease but did not provide conclusive results.[23–25] In an experimental study conducted by Niang and colleagues,[25] it was demonstrated that treatment with oxytetracycline did not result in significant sequestra formation in CBPP-infected animals, suggesting that CBPP treatment with long-acting-oxytetracycline does not increase the number of carriers. In a similar study, Ottina and colleagues[23] showed that treatment of CBPP-infected cattle with oxytetracycline lowered the severity of the clinical signs of the disease. While these results still need to be confirmed under field conditions, at present, an effective vaccination policy remains the only realistic method of choice for control of the disease in countries where CBPP is endemic.[12]

CONTROL CHALLENGES IN AFRICA

Many efforts have been made to effectively control CBPP in Africa with varying degrees of success. These include several successive coordinated programs such as the Joint Project 16 (JP 16) in the 1970s, and the Pan African Control for Epizootics (PACE). These programs supported CBPP control through a policy of compulsory mass vaccination campaigns in the endemic areas of Africa, followed by quarantines, test and slaughter with compensation for infected cattle, and disease outbreak reporting. Furthermore, a combined control effort for rinderpest and CBPP was jointly conducted during the Pan African Rinderpest Campaigns (PARC), in which vaccine containing both rinderpest virus strain and CBPP attenuated vaccine strain T1/SR (Bisec) was used. This approach enabled the eradication of rinderpest and contributed to the efficient control of CBPP. Following the 1996/1997 cessation of joint vaccination, because of the successful rinderpest eradication program, there has been a resurgence of CBPP in many countries despite continuation of vaccination campaigns using T1/44 CBPP vaccine.[18]

The challenges of CBPP control in sub-Saharan African countries are well documented.[4,10,21] They are all related in part to the decline of funding in public veterinary services following the imposed structural adjustment programs in the 1980s. These have resulted in a decline in the enforcement of animal health policies by the veterinary authorities and consequently poor implementation of CBPP surveillance and control programs in endemic areas.

The current situation in many infected sub-Saharan countries is characterized by

- Uncoordinated and unsustainable vaccination programs,
- Uncontrolled movement of cattle associated with pastoral livelihood practices,
- Misuse of antibiotics in the treatment of respiratory diseases (including CBPP) by farmers,
- Limited or no access to quality CBPP vaccines,
- Low vaccination coverage, and
- Dependence on external funding to support CBPP vaccination programs.

These factors are compounded by civil unrest and climate-related constraints in some areas. The absence of a compensation policy for cattle destroyed as a result of CBPP outbreaks is also a disincentive for CBPP outbreak reporting. Consequently, CBPP still persists in many sub-Saharan African countries with increasing incidence in some of them, resurgence in previously infected countries, and the perceived threats of spread to hitherto disease-free countries (eg, Northern and Southern African countries) in the continent.

Efforts should be made within limited resources to train veterinary staff in disease surveillance and performing abattoir/slaughter facilities inspection, as this method is cheap and effective in surveillance for the disease. Training of field staff is encouraged for CBPP vaccination campaigns to ensure maintenance of cold chain in the field and proper inoculation techniques. Countries in Africa affected by CBPP and other

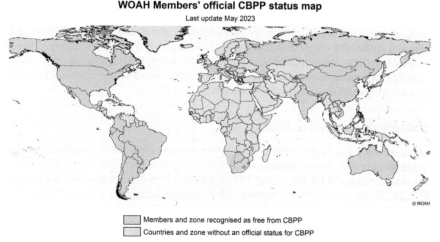

WOAH Members' official CBPP status map
Last update May 2023

☐ Members and zone recognised as free from CBPP
☐ Countries and zone without an official status for CBPP

Fig. 4. Countries officially recognized free from CBPP by WOAH. (World Organisation for Animal Health (WOAH) (2023). - WAHIS Official Disease Status. Retrieved from https://www. woah.org/en/what-we-do/animal-health-and-welfare/official-disease-status/. Screenshot or copy by Elsevier. Reproduced with permission. The World Organisation for Animal Health (WOAH) bears no responsibility for the integrity or accuracy of the data contained herein, but not limited to, any deletion, manipulation, or reformatting of data that may have occurred beyond its control.)

transboundary animal diseases (TADs) should consider establishing livestock insurance schemes to serve as a 'cushion" for losses during outbreaks of CBPP and other TADs.

WORLD ORGANISATION FOR ANIMAL HEALTH DISEASE-FREE STATUS

CBPP is one of the six diseases for which currently WOAH has established an official procedure for recognition of disease-free status for trade purposes. A member country wishing to be officially recognized as CBPP free by WOAH can apply following the guidelines and steps laid out in Chapter 1.6. of the WOAH Terrestrial Code and comply with all requirements specified for CBPP.[6] Countries or zones currently officially recognized free from CBPP by WOAH are shown in **Fig. 4.** The United States, Canada, and Mexico all are officially recognized as free. WOAH also offers a procedure for Members engaged in CBPP control to apply for official recognition of their disease control program in accordance with the provisions of the Terrestrial Code.[6]

In sub-Saharan Africa where the disease is endemic, only 4 countries are currently recognized as officially free (see **Fig. 4**) from CBPP by WOAH, that is, Botswana, Eswatini, South Africa (country-wide), and Namibia (zone located south of the Veterinary Cordon Fence). Namibia and Zambia are also the only countries having a WOAH-endorsed official control program for CBPP. Many other countries are free from the disease, although they might not have sought official freedom from the disease from WOAH.[26]

SUMMARY

CBPP is a classic example of a TAD requiring regional efforts and active cooperation among neighboring countries for its effective prevention and control. Although its exact distribution, incidence, and impact have not been well established, the disease is known to be endemic in sub-Saharan Africa, where it has a severe socio-economic impact by affecting peoples' livelihoods and general well-being. Economic stagnation in many affected countries has prevented progressive control of the disease, which compromises continental and global eradication. Elimination of the disease in infected countries or regions can be achieved by combined control measures and effective control of animal movements. The strategic approach to CBPP disease management should be based on progressive control leading ultimately to area-wide freedom from the infection. Existing tools can be used for a successful coordinated control program when applied appropriately. A CBPP control program could be used as a basis for the improvement of veterinary services, especially in respect of surveillance, control, public-private partnership, and regional coordination.

The persistence of the disease in Africa represents a constant threat to other parts of the world. All countries free from CBPP should have emergency response plans with measures to prevent introduction of CBPP from neighboring countries or zones. These plans should include means for rapid confirmation, both in the field and in the laboratory, as well as a rapid intervention strategy in line with WOAH requirements.

There is a need for national governments, private stakeholders, regional bodies, international intergovernmental organizations, and funding partners to invest in CBPP control as a basis for improving food security, people's livelihoods, and general well-being, therefore contributing to achieving Sustainable Development Goals.

DISCLOSURE

The author(s) declared no potential conflicts of interest with respect to the research, authorship, and/or publication of this article.

REFERENCES

1. USDA. Contagious bovine pleuropneumonia standard operating procedures: 1. Overview of etiology and ecology. 2017 (updated in 2022). Available at: https://www.aphis.usda.gov/animal_health/emergency_management/downloads/sop/cbpp-fadprep-ee.pdf. [Accessed 20 October 2023].
2. Tambi NE, Maina WO, Ndi C. An estimation of the economic impact of contagious bovine pleuropneumonia in Africa. Rev sci tech Off int Epiz 2006;25(3):999–1012. Available at: https://doc.woah.org/dyn/portal/index.xhtml?page=alo&aloId=30609. [Accessed 20 October 2023].
3. Lefèvre PC. Contagious bovine pleuropneumonia. In: Lefevre PC, Blancou J, Chermette R, et al, editors. Infectious and parasitic diseases of livestock: bacterial diseases, fungal diseases, parasitic diseases, Volume 2, PART 3: bacterial diseases, 66). Paris: Lavoisier; 2011. p. 791–809.
4. Alhaji NB, Idoko A, Terhemba Ikpa L, et al. Contagious Bovine Pleuropneumonia: Challenges and Prospects Regarding Diagnosis and Control Strategies in Africa. Vet Med (Auckl) 2020;11:71–85. Available at: https://doi.org/10.2147/VMRR.S180025 [Accessed 20 October 2023].
5. Amanfu W. Contagious Bovine Pleuropneumonia. In: Kardjadj M, Diallo A, Lancelot R, editors. Transboundary animal diseases in Sahelian Africa and connected regions. Cham: Springer; 2019. p. 423–37.
6. WOAH. Contagious bovine Pleuropneumonia. 2023. Available at: https://www.woah.org/en/disease/contagious-bovine-pleuropneumonia/#ui-id-2. [Accessed 20 October 2023].
7. FAO. Control Of contagious bovine pleuropneumonia - a policy for coordinated actions. FAO animal production and health paper 180. Rome: FAO; 2019.

Available at: https://www.fao.org/documents/card/en/c/CA3949EN. [Accessed 20 October 2023].

8. WOAH disease card. Contagious bovine pleuropneumonia. 2020. Available at: https://www.woah.org/en/document/contagious_bovine_pleuropneumonia/. [Accessed 20 October 2023].

9. Di Teodoro G, Marruchella G, Di Provvido A, et al. Contagious Bovine Pleuropneumonia: A Comprehensive Overview. Veterinary Pathology 2020;57(4): 476–89.

10. Amanfu W. Contagious bovine pleuropneumonia (Lungsickness) in Africa. Onderstepoort J Vet Res 2009;76:13–7. Available at: https://www.scielo.org.za/pdf/ojvr/v76n1/05.pdf. [Accessed 20 October 2023].

11. Abera Z, Mengistu D, Batu G, et al. Review on Contagious Bovine Pleuropneumonia and its Economic Impacts. Acad J Anim Dis 2016;5(1):01–15. Available at: https://www.idosi.org/ajad/6(2)17/4.pdf. [Accessed 20 October 2023].

12. FAO. CBPP Round Table: Can CBPP be eradicated? FAO-OIE-AU/IBAR-IAEA Consultative group on CBPP Fifth meeting, Rome, 14-16 2015. FAO animal production and health proceedings No. 19. FAO; 2016. Available at: https://www.fao.org/publications/card/fr/c/ac99131d-a342-4bfb-b8b2-c850406fb1ee/. [Accessed 20 October 2023].

13. Demil E. Review on economic impact of contagious bovine pleuropneumonia (CBPP). Acad J Anim Dis 2017;6(2):51–6. Available at: https://www.idosi.org/ajad/6(2)17/4.pdf. [Accessed 20 October 2023].

14. Masiga WN, Domenech J, Windsor RS. Manifestation and epidemiology of contagious bovine pleuropneumonia in Africa. Rev Sci Tech 1996;15(4):1283–308.

15. Recognizing FAO. Contagious bovine pleuropneumonia (revised edition). Rome: FAO; 2002. p. 32pp. Available at: https://www.fao.org/3/Y4142E/Y4142E00.htm. [Accessed 20 October 2023].

16. Newton LG, Norris R. Clearing a continent: the eradication of bovine pleuropneumonia from Australia. Collingwood, Australia: CSIRO Publishing; 2000.

17. Marobela-Roborokgwe C. Contagious bovine pleuropneumonia in Botswana: experience with control, eradication, prevention and surveillance. Vet Ital 2011; 47(4):397–405.

18. Thiaucourt F, Nwankpa ND, Amanfu W. Contagious Bovine Pleuropneumonia. In: Metwally S, Viljoen G, El Idrissi A, editors. Veterinary vaccines: principles and applications. First Edition. John Wiley & Sons Ltd and FAO; 2021. p. 317–26. Available at: https://www.fao.org/documents/card/en/c/cc2031en. [Accessed 20 October 2023].

19. Thiaucourt F, Yaya A, Wesonga H, et al. Contagious bovine pleuropneumonia. A reassessment of the efficacy of vaccines used in Africa. Ann N Y Acad Sci 2003; 916:71–80. Available at: https://doi.org/10.1111/j.1749-6632.2000.tb05276.x [Accessed 20 October 2023].

20. FAO. CBPP Control: Antibiotics to the Rescue? FAO-OIE-AU/IBARIAEA Consultative Group Meeting on CBPP in Africa. Rome, 6-8 2006. FAO animal production and health proceedings No. 8. FAO; 2006. 129. Available at: https://www.fao.org/3/ah672e/ah672e.pdf. [Accessed 20 October 2023].

21. Towards FAO. Sustainable CBPP Control Programmes for Africa. FAO-OIE-AU/IBAR-IAEA Consultative Group on Contagious Bovine Pleuropneumonia Third Meeting, . FAO animal production and health proceedings No. 3. Rome: FAO; 2004. Available at: www.fao.org/3/y5510e/y5510e00.htm. [Accessed 20 October 2023].

22. Mariner JC, Catley A. The dynamics of CBPP endemism and development of effective control strategies. In: Towards sustainable CBPP control programmes for Africa. FAO-OIE-AU/IBAR-IAEA consultative group on contagious bovine pleuropneumonia third meeting. FAO animal production and health proceedings No. 3. Rome: FAO; 2004. Available at: https://www.fao.org/3/y5510e/y5510e0e.htm#bm14. [Accessed 20 October 2023].

23. Otina B, Kitala P, Bebora L, et al. Effects of Long Acting Oxytetracycline on Contagious Bovine Pleuropneumonia Experimentally Infected Cattle. Tanzan J Sci 2022;48(4):954–61. Available at: https://doi.org/10.4314/tjs.v48i4.20 [Accessed 20 October 2023].

24. Muuka GM, Songolo A, Kabilika S, et al. Observations of oxytetracycline treatment effects in a contagious bovine pleuropneumonia naturally infected herd in Zambia. J. Vet. Sci. Anim. Health 2017;9(6):110–5.

25. Niang M, Sery A, Doucoure M, et al. Experimental studies on the effect of long-acting oxytetracycline treatment in the development of sequestra in contagious bovine pleuropneumonia-infected cattle. Journal of Veterinary Medicine and Animal Health 2010;2(4):35–45. Available at: https://academicjournals.org/article/article1379428705_Niang%20et%20al.pdf. [Accessed 20 October 2023].

26. FAO, WOAH, AU-IBAR. GF-TADs for Africa Contagious bovine pleuropneumonia (CBPP) Standing Group of Experts (SGE) for Africa. Inaugural meeting 6 – 15 June 2023. Report of the online event. WOAH and FAO. 2023. Available at: https://rr-africa.woah.org/wp-content/uploads/2023/06/report-v3-english-vfinal.pdf. [Accessed 20 October 2023].

Rift Valley Fever

J. Brian Kimble, PhD[a], Leela Noronha, DVM, PhD[a],
Jessie D. Trujillo, DVM, PhD[b], Dana Mitzel, PhD[a],
Juergen A. Richt, DVM, PhD[b,c], William C. Wilson, PhD[a,*]

KEYWORDS

- Rift valley fever • Abortion • Hemorrhagic fever • Sheep • Goats • Cattle

KEY POINTS

- Rift Valley fever (RVF) is a viral disease of domestic ruminants and wild hooved animals of Africa and the Middle East but can also infect humans.
- RVF virus is spread by several species of mosquitoes and causes intermittent outbreaks.
- Predominantly found in Sub-Saharan Africa, confirmed outbreaks in nearby island nations and the Arabian Peninsula highlight the increasing geographic footprint in endemic regions.
- Animal outbreaks are associated with high rates of abortions, neonatal die-offs, and influenza-like illness to occasionally lethal disease in people.
- RVF is primarily a febrile disease that mainly involves the liver.

Rift Valley fever (RVF) is a zoonotic viral disease that affects domestic and wild ruminants such as cattle, sheep, goats, camels, and buffaloes. Rift Valley fever phlebovirus (RVFV), the causative agent of RVF, can also infect humans. RVFV is an arthropod-borne virus (arbovirus) that is primarily spread through the bites of infected mosquitoes. RVFV was first isolated and characterized in the Rift Valley of Kenya in 1931 and is endemic throughout sub-Saharan Africa, including Comoros and Madagascar, the Arabian Peninsula (Saudi Arabia and Yemen), and Mayotte.[1] Highlighting the transboundary nature of RVFV was the first non-African outbreak that occurred in Saudi Arabia and Yemen in 2000 and various serologic surveys that revealed its potential expansion to additional African and Middle Eastern countries.[2] Disease prevention in animals is best facilitated by vaccination, vector control programs, and restrictions on livestock movement during outbreaks.

VIROLOGY

RVFV is a member of the genus *Phlebovirus* in the *Phenuiviridae* family of the Bunya-virales order (reviewed in Ref[3]). Like most bunyaviruses, RVFV is an arbovirus, that is

[a] Foreign Arthropod-Borne Animal Diseases Research Unit, National Bio and Agro-Defense Facility, USDA, ARS, Manhattan, KS, USA; [b] Diganostic Medicine/Pathobiology, Kansas State University, Manhattan, KS, USA; [c] Department of Veterinary Tropical Diseases, Faculty of Veterinary Science, University of Pretoria, Onderstepoort, South Africa
* Corresponding author. Foreign Arthropod-Borne Animal Diseases Research Unit, National Bio and Agro-Defense Facility, P.O. Box 1807, Manhattan, KS 66505.
E-mail address: william.wilson2@usda.gov

Vet Clin Food Anim 40 (2024) 293–304
https://doi.org/10.1016/j.cvfa.2024.01.004
0749-0720/24/Published by Elsevier Inc.

a virus transmitted by arthropods, specifically *Aedes* and *Culex spp.* mosquitoes. The virus has a tripartite, single-stranded, negative/ambisense RNA genome consisting of the L, M, and S segments (large, medium, and small, respectively; **Fig. 1**). The viral RNA associates with the RNA-dependent RNA-polymerase L protein (encoded on the L segment) and the nucleoprotein N (encoded on the S segment) to form the ribonucleoprotein complex. After the completion of replication, RVF viral particles assemble and bud from the Golgi apparatus; the viral particles are enveloped by host-derived membranes containing the viral glycoproteins Gn and Gc (encoded both on the M segment). The Gn and Gc surface glycoproteins are responsible for virus attachment and host cell entry which allows the release of the viral genetic material into the cytoplasm. RVFV expresses other viral proteins such as the 78 kDa protein (encoded on the M segment), important for mosquito infection, or the nonstructural NSs and NSm proteins (encoded on the S and M segment, respectively), important for modulizations of the host cell environment (NSm) and host immune response (NSs).

EPIDEMIOLOGY

RVFV infections cause disease in domestic and wild ruminants across Africa and parts of the Middle East. Humans living close to livestock are at risk for infection with this zoonotic pathogen.[4–6] Besides sheep, goats, cattle, and camels, RVF is also found in wildlife such as buffalo and springbok; seroepidemiology also identified other susceptible African wildlife species[7] including various rodent species.[8] The potential role of wildlife in RVFV epidemiology is not well understood, especially with regard to North America; however, white-tail deer have been shown to be experimentally susceptible to infection, disease, and transmission of RVFV.[9] Transmission of the virus to mammals is primarily caused via the feeding of infected mosquitoes. Numerous species of mosquitoes from 7 different genera have been shown to be competent for infection and transmission of RVFV, either naturally or in lab settings.[10] Outbreaks of RVF occur unpredictably at 5 to 35 year intervals and are most often associated with heavy seasonal rainfall and flooding, which are conditions ideal for the hatching of mosquito eggs and mosquito breeding.[11] During interepidemic periods, the virus can be maintained by vertical transovarial transmission of RVFV from infected female *Aedes spp.*

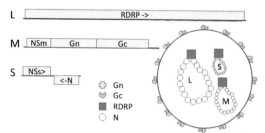

Fig. 1. Schematic of RVFV virion and genome structure. Viral RNA is wrapped around the nucleoprotein N (*circles*) and forms a loop structure with the RNA-dependent RNA polymerase L (RDRP, *blue square*). Gn (*green cross*) and Gc (*green pie*) are embedded in the host-derived virus envelope that packages the 3 RNA segments L, M, and S. The L (6.4 kb), M (3.9 kb), and S (1.7 kb) segments encode 8 viral proteins. The RDRP is the only protein produced from the L segment. The M segment encodes the 2 surface glycoproteins Gn and Gc. Alternate start codons within the M segment are utilized to produce the NSm, NSm′, and the 78 kDa protein. The S segment is an ambisense RNA that produces the NSs and N proteins.

mosquitoes to eggs and the resultant adult mosquitoes.[12] This is possible because desiccated eggs of some mosquito species can remain infectious for months to years, depending on the conditions. Transovarial transmission has also been demonstrated experimentally in *Culex tarsalis*.[13] Other, yet undetermined, mechanisms for RVFV maintenance in the environment may also play a role. Serologic surveys indicate that low levels of livestock and wildlife infections may support the existence of undetected transmission during interepidemic periods.[14]

RVF disease was likely first reported in 1912 but the virus was not isolated until 1930 during an outbreak in Tanzania and Kenya[2]; however, molecular epidemiology suggests that the virus has been present in Africa since the late 1800s.[15–17] The presence of RVFV has been confirmed by viral isolation or serologic surveys in countries in Africa, nearby island nations, and the Arabian Peninsula.[1] Serologic surveys of livestock and humans have identified antibodies to RVFV in additional countries, indicating that the virus could be more widespread; this warrants surveillance for RVFV outside of known endemic areas (**Fig. 2**).[2,5] RVFV is not found in North or South America; however, US mosquito species have been shown to be competent vectors.[18]

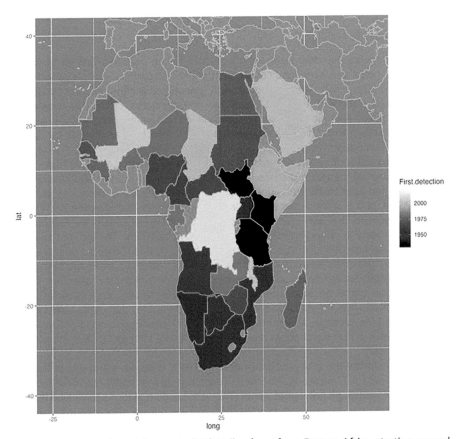

Fig. 2. Temporal and spatial spread of Rift Valley fever from Eastern Africa, starting around 1930. Map of combined serologic and virological evidence of RVFV presence across Africa and the Middle East. Colors indicate first year of evidence; color code from earlier (~1930; *dark*) to later (2000s; *light*) years. Map based on data from the CDC.[1]

TRANSMISSION CYCLE

Vertebrate hosts can be infected though the bite of infected mosquitoes or by exposure to blood or tissues of infected animals. Mosquito-borne transmission is the most likely infection pathway for livestock. Initial targets of infection are thought to be tissue-resident macrophages and other antigen-presenting cells.[19] These cells carry the virus to local draining lymph nodes and amplify the infection, causing viremia (infectious virus in the blood) and viral spread to the primary sites of replication: the liver and the spleen.[20,21] Viremia can occur between 2 and 4 days postexposure and can last up to 7 days. The fetus and neonate animals are highly susceptible to RVFV infection and can develop viremia in as little as 12 to 36 hours. Once an animal is viremic, it can pass RVFV to a naïve mosquito via blood feeding and the transmission cycle restarts. Another important route of infection is contact exposure to infected tissues and body fluids. This route of infection often occurs in people with close contact to livestock such as butchers, farmers, and veterinarians taking care of sick animals, often during abortion storms. Although there are no reports of infections from exposure to raw milk, reports indicate milk samples from susceptible animal species have tested positive for RVFV-specific RNA; also, there is a strong association between consuming or collecting raw milk and RVFV seroconversion.[22–24]

CLINICAL DISEASE

Disease susceptibility decreases with age and varies between animal species.[25] Sheep and goats are more susceptible than cattle and camels, and there are differences in susceptibility across breed and genotype within livestock species.[26] Neonatal lambs and kids less than 1 week old are highly susceptible. The relative susceptibility of wild animals has not been established. Experimentally, white-tailed deer have been shown to be highly susceptible to RVFV infection resulting in clinical disease and virus transmission.[9]

   Most livestock outbreaks are usually associated with high incidence of abortions (abortion storms), newborn die-offs, and spill-over into the human population. RVFV infections can lead to clinical signs ranging from inapparent to peracute. Newborn lambs, kids, and to a lesser extent, calves, develop severe liver disease with high fevers, listlessness, and abdominal pain. Icterus (common in calves) has also been reported. Mortality in young animals varies from 70% to 100%. The incubation period can be as short as 12 hours postexposure but is typically 24 to 36 hours postexposure. Older sheep and goats develop clinical signs 24 to 72 hours postexposure that include fever, anorexia, listlessness, diarrhea, and icterus with a mortality rate from 10% to 30%.[27] Adult cattle develop anorexia, diarrhea, dysgalactia, excessive salivation, and nasal discharge. Clinical signs are often not apparent in adult cattle, and mortality is less than 10%. Viremia, an important factor in the transmission cycle of RVFV, lasts for 1 to 3 days in less susceptible breeds, but can be as long as 10 days in more susceptible ones.[27]

   Abortion storms are a key indicator of large RVFV outbreaks and cause the main economic impact in livestock. Abortion rates typically reach 90% to 100% in sheep and goats.[27] Although not well studied, RVF-associated abortions have also been reported in camels and African buffalo.[28,29] RVFV-induced abortions may also be associated with increased maternal mortality.[30] Vertical transmission to the fetus in utero typically targets the liver and brain of the fetus; in utero infection can result in necrotizing viral placentitis resulting in abortion prior to fetal infection.[31] Thus, a failure to identify RVFV or RVFV RNA in fetal tissues does not rule out RVF as an etiology.

There exists a complex symptomatology of RFVF infection in humans, many of which are nonspecific.[32] RVFV infections in humans commonly present as self-limiting influenza-like febrile illness that can last 3 to 4 days but may recrudesce and last for up to 10 days. Viremia can be detected for 3 to 4 days during the febrile stage of the disease. The overall human mortality rate is estimated at less than 1%.[33] Occasionally, a macular rash, jaundice, and bleeding may occur, which is indicative of RVFV-associated hemorrhagic fever, usually with fatal outcome.[34,35] Additionally, some patients develop hepatic necrosis or ocular disease resulting in partial or total blindness, while some develop encephalitis with neurologic signs including neck rigidity, limb weakness, confusion, hyperreflexia, and coma.[36,37] Vision loss and neurologic symptoms can be temporal or permanent and may present in the same patient.[38]

PATHOGENESIS

Severe RVF disease is mainly observed in neonatal lambs and kids while cattle and older sheep and goats exhibit milder disease. The most prominent pathologic features of an RVFV infection in ruminants are small, necrotic lesions (1–3 mm size) in the liver (**Fig. 3**).[39] These lesions can vary in density from multifocal liver foci to coalescing necrotic foci in more severe cases. A peracute infection results in an enlarged, friable, and discolored brown-orange liver with accentuated lobulation.[25,40] Gall bladder involvement is often seen with notable edema and hemorrhage in the gall bladder wall and blood in the luminal space.[41] Lymph nodes and kidneys can be enlarged and edematous with petechial hemorrhages; the spleen is also often enlarged and congested.[39] Diffuse pulmonary congestion is often noted. Hemorrhages on the inner and outer surfaces of the heart and on serosal surfaces can be observed.

Microscopically, liver lesions are characterized by multifocal to coalescing, midzonal to periportal necrosis of hepatocytes, accompanied by variable hemorrhages and inflammation (**Fig. 4**). Necrotic foci consist of well-defined foci with loss of architecture and hepatic cords. Hepatocyte drop-out, hepatic swelling and karyorrhexis, as well as cellular lysis and apoptotic cells (councilman-like bodies) are mixed with fibrin and hemorrhage and cellular and nuclear debris. Often there are infiltrates of neutrophils, macrophages, and lymphocytes within and surrounding necrotic foci.[40] Mixed periportal infiltrates of inflammatory cells and fibrin thrombi in vessels can also occur. Necrotic foci are of varying size, can coalesce and affect entire liver lobes in severe

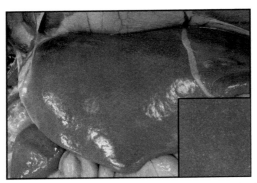

Fig. 3. Liver from a calf experimentally infected with wild-type RVFV displaying typical pathologic lesions. Liver *in situ* with 1 to 3 mm pale, necrotic foci (highlighted in *insert*), accompanied by mild generalized liver enlargement with rounded edges, and slight pallor.

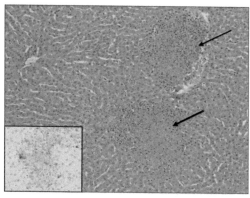

Fig. 4. Microscopic hepatic lesions due to RVFV infection. Multiple areas of parenchymal necrosis occur in centrilobular zone or adjacent to central veins. Black arrows denote necrotic foci; the upper lesion contains infiltrates of lymphocytes (40x). Inset: Immunohistochemical staining for RVFV antigen present at the edge of the necrotic lesions (100X).

cases.[25] In some instances, acidophilic intranuclear inclusion bodies are appreciated.[41] When performing ultrastructural analysis, RVFV-infected cells, mainly in fetal and neonate samples, display filamentous intranuclear bodies consisting of the viral NSs protein.[42] Immunohistochemistry (IHC) using RVFV-specific hyperimmune serum/antibodies is used to confirm the presence of RVFV-specific antigen in infected livers. IHC-positive cells are commonly located at the periphery of necrotic lesions (see **Fig. 4**); however, in fulminant RVF infections, IHC staining can occur throughout the entire hepatic parenchyma.[41]

DIAGNOSIS

RVFV infections in humans usually present as influenza-like illness accompanied by hepatic disease and/or hemorrhaging, whereas infections in domestic ruminants are usually accompanied by abortion storms and neonatal deaths. RVF is characterized by hepatic lesions seen during macroscopic and histopathological examinations. Differential diagnoses from other conditions causing hemorrhagic disease with liver necrosis and death include bacterial septicemia, plant or chemical toxicosis, and other hemorrhagic viral diseases. Laboratory confirmation of the presence of antigen, viral RNA, and/or RVFV-specific antibodies should be made for definitive diagnosis.

Diagnostic specimens should include sera and anticoagulated whole blood from live animals or samples of liver, spleen, lymph nodes, kidneys, and/or heart from dead animals and aborted fetuses. Also, placenta is useful in some instances if *postmortem* autolysis is not too advanced. Fetal tissue is often autolyzed, leading to the degradation of viral antigens and genomic RNA material as well as poor tissue morphology. Appropriate personal protective equipment (PPE) should be worn when performing *postmortem* examinations and tissue collections. Samples should be handled with the assumption of the presence of infectious RVFV and executed under enhanced BSL-3 conditions.[43] Samples should be sent to appropriate governmental reference laboratories at 4°C or frozen and in accordance with biological hazard regulations.

RVFV can be isolated from serum, plasma, anticoagulated blood, or from various organs/tissues using susceptible cell lines such as Vero, BHK, or AP61 cells.[44] Virus-positive cell cultures are identified by the presence of cytopathic effects with confirmatory IHC staining or reverse transcriptase polymerase chain reaction (RT-PCR). RVFV antigen detection is primarily done by enzyme-linked immunosorbent assay (ELISA) which can detect RVF viral proteins in blood and tissues or by IHC staining on formalin-fixed, paraffin-embedded (FFPE) tissues. Viral RNA can be detected in FFPE tissues via in situ hybridization or RT-PCR.[45] Lateral flow devices have proven to be effective and are in development but are not yet currently commercially available. Viral genomic components can be detected by RT-PCR while quantitative real-time RT-PCR is able to quantify viral genome copies, a useful tool in tracking disease stage and progression. There are numerous *in-house* protocols and commercial kits available for either ELISA or RT-PCR, and the World Organisation for Animal Health (formerly OIE) has a collection of protocols which are utilized by reference labs worldwide.[43,44] Viral isolation, antigen detection, and RT-PCR are useful when virus is present (2–4 days postexposure in blood and up to 8 days in tissues). Detection of RVFV infection after the initial exposure/replication period is accomplished via serologic assays for RVFV antibody detection. RVFV antibody detection is primarily done by ELISA using recombinant N or other viral proteins as antigen. ELISAs can differentiate between IgM (early antibodies) and IgG (long-term antibodies) antibodies. Indirect immunofluorescence using RVFV-infected cells or infected tissue slides can also be used. Neutralization tests (NTs) are also commonly used; they are cell culture-based assays that test a serum sample's ability to block viral infection (virus neutralization assay) or reduce the number of viral plaques formed (plaque reduction NT).

PREVENTION AND CONTROL

Owing to the sporadic nature of RVFV outbreaks and the unpredictability of heavy rain/flooding, vector control and the movement of livestock to drier areas is not an effective mitigation strategy. The most effective solutions within endemic areas are regular vaccination of highly susceptible livestock and restriction of livestock movement from affected areas to nonaffected areas. Surveillance of susceptible livestock and wildlife near outbreak locations and in areas between endemic and nonendemic regions is important to determine whether control efforts are working and for confirming the onset of outbreaks. The potential movement of RVFV into nonendemic countries via legal and illegal movement of animals, mosquito vectors, and humans has been recently reviewed.[18] Community outreach and educational programs are critical to support the above-mentioned mitigation strategies.

Currently, only a few RVFV vaccines are licensed for veterinary use; there is no human vaccine available. Thus, proper PPE such as latex or vinyl gloves, face masks (minimally surgical masks but preferably N95 or power-assisted purified air respirators), scrubs or coveralls, and boots should be worn, if RVFV is suspected. The most commonly used vaccine in the endemic area in Africa is the Smithburn vaccine, which is a live attenuated vaccine produced from an RVFV isolate derived from a mosquito pool in Uganda; this RVFV isolate was passed more than 100 times in mouse brains.[46] The vaccine is inexpensive, can be produced easily, and provides robust, long-lasting immunity from a single dose application. However, it is not recommended for certain animal species and pregnant animals as it causes abortion and teratogenic effects.[47,48] Like most live attenuated vaccines, there are concerns of reversion to virulence or reassortment with wild-type RVF viruses.[49] Therefore, the Smithburn vaccine is only recommended for use in endemic areas. The live attenuated Clone 13 RVFV vaccine has been increasingly used across Africa in the past 10 years after licensure in South Africa.[49] Clone 13 is naturally attenuated and produces a protective and long-lasting immune response similar to the Smithburn vaccine; in addition, it is safe to use in pregnant animals when applied as directed on the label.[50] One study showed that an overdose of Clone 13 in pregnant sheep resulted in stillbirths and malformed fetuses; thus, following the label recommendations for the Clone 13 vaccine dose is critically important.[51] The MP-12 RVFV vaccine is another live attenuated vaccine that is conditionally licensed in the United States and Canada for emergency use. The MP-12 vaccine induces robust and long-term immunity and has been shown to be safe and efficacious.[52] However, a cell-passaged MP-12 vaccine was shown to induce teratogenic effects when administered to pregnant animals.[53]

Additional next-generation RVFV vaccines are in development. These include subunit vaccines, vectored vaccines such as a chimp adenovirus vectored vaccine, and a 4 segmented altered genome vaccine.[54,55] Subunit vaccines are safe and offer the capability of differentiating infected from vaccinated animals (DIVA) when paired with the appropriate diagnostic testing platform (eg, DIVA ELISA). Subunit vaccines currently under development require 2 vaccination doses to be efficacious. Although DIVA compatible subunit RVFV vaccines are of value in nonendemic countries; there are concerns for their usefulness in sub-Saharan Africa where nomadic herding practices are used and multi-dose vaccines regimens would be impractical. The hot climate and limited infrastructure and resources of endemic regions in the Africa/Arabian Peninsula make vaccine stability and storage conditions important considerations as well. Other vaccine strategies such as DNA or mRNA vaccines are currently being investigated and may result in novel vaccine platforms.[56]

SUMMARY

RVFV is an arbovirus endemic to much of the African continent. RVF outbreaks have also occurred in the Comoros Island, Madagascar, Mayotte, and the Arabian Peninsula. The virus is maintained during interepidemic periods in *Aedes* mosquitoes via transovarial transmission and through low-level RVFV infections of livestock and wildlife species. Large outbreaks occur sporadically during periods of heavy rainfall and persistent flooding with the emergence of infected mosquitoes breeding in floodwater. A multitude of different mosquito genera and species are competent vectors for RVFV replication and transmission. Sheep, goats, cattle, and camels are susceptible livestock species, and the virus has been also isolated from wild African buffalo and springbok. In domestic livestock, susceptibility dependent on species, age, and breed. RVFV is a zoonotic pathogen and human cases often accompany livestock outbreaks. The Americas are free of RVF, so vigilant veterinary practitioners are key for first raising concern of a potential introduction.

Outbreaks in livestock are generally recognized by abortion storms and increased neonatal deaths and flu-like symptoms in humans. The virus causes hepatitis and must be differentiated from other hepatic diseases by virus isolation, antigen detection, RT-PCR methods, or by serology. Veterinary practitioners should contact their state and/or federal animal health official should they suspect an unusual disease outbreak. This is especially important as infected humans may develop hemorrhagic disease, or ocular or neurologic signs that can be fatal. Currently, there is no human RVFV vaccine available. In contrast, live attenuated RVFV vaccines are available for livestock in endemic areas and are the best tools for disease control. These live attenuated RVFV vaccines are highly effective but are not safe for use in pregnant animals. Continued improvement of vaccine strategies with the implementation of novel technologies resulting in a safe and DIVA-compatible RVFV vaccine that induces a rapid and long-lasting immunity with a single dose is critical and may allow for improved prevention and control strategies in the future.

CLINICS CARE POINTS

- Animals infected with RVFV present clinical symptoms ranging from inapparent to peracute. Indicators include high herd abortion rates and newborn mortality, severe liver disease, fevers, and abdominal pain.

- Zoonotic infections of humans can occur after mosquito bites or handling of infectious animal fluids or tissues during veterinary care or butchering. People present with febrile illness that can progress in severity to include hepatic disease, hemorrhagic fever, neurologic involvement, or death.

- Diagnostic samples from suspected cases should be handled under enhanced BSL3 conditions. Definitive diagnostic tests include viral isolation, antigen detection, RT-PCR, and pathogen-specific antibody detection.

- A few vaccines are regionally approved, but current options using live attenuted vaccines have significant drawbacks. Recent advances offer hope for better vaccine options. Outbreak control is achieved by restricting the movement of susceptible animals into or out of affected areas.

DISCLOSURE

Mention of trade names or commercial products in this publication is solely for the purpose of providing specific information and does not imply recommendation or endorsement by the U.S. Department of Agriculture (USDA). The conclusions in this report are those of the authors and do not necessarily represent the views of the USDA. The USDA is an equal opportunity provider and employer.

FUNDING

This work was funded in part by the USDA, Agricultural Research Service and by the US Department of Homeland Security Center of Excellence for Emerging and Zoonotic Animal Diseases (CEEZAD), Grant No. 2010-ST061-AG0001, and NBAF Transition Funds from the State of Kansas. Funding for this study was also partially provided through the AMP and MCB Cores of the Center of Emerging and Zoonotic Infectious Diseases (CEZID) from the National Institute of General Medical Sciences (NIGMS) under Award Number P20GM130448.

REFERENCES

1. CDC. RVF distribution map. 2023. Available at: https://www.cdc.gov/vhf/rvf/outbreaks/distribution-map.html.
2. Bron GM, Strimbu K, Cecilia H, et al. Over 100 Years of Rift Valley Fever: A Patchwork of Data on Pathogen Spread and Spillover. Pathogens 2021;10(6).
3. Nair N, Osterhaus ADME, Rimmelzwaan GF, et al. Rift Valley Fever Virus-Infection, Pathogenesis and Host Immune Responses. Pathogens 2023;12(9).
4. Johnson SAM, Asmah R, Awuni JA, et al. Evidence of Rift Valley Fever Virus Circulation in Livestock and Herders in Southern Ghana. Viruses 2023;15(6).
5. Clark MHA, Warimwe GM, Di Nardo A, et al. Systematic literature review of Rift Valley fever virus seroprevalence in livestock, wildlife and humans in Africa from 1968 to 2016. PLoS Neglected Trop Dis 2018;12(7):e0006627.
6. Sang R, Kioko E, Lutomiah J, et al. Rift Valley fever virus epidemic in Kenya, 2006/2007: the entomologic investigations. Am J Trop Med Hyg 2010;83(2 Suppl):28–37.

7. Capobianco Dondona A, Aschenborn O, Pinoni C, et al. Rift Valley Fever Virus among Wild Ruminants, Etosha National Park, Namibia, 2011. Emerg Infect Dis 2016;22(1):128–30.

8. Rostal MK, Liang JE, Zimmermann D, et al. Rift Valley Fever: Does Wildlife Play a Role? ILAR J 2017;58(3):359–70.

9. Wilson WC, Kim IJ, Trujillo JD, et al. Susceptibility of White-Tailed Deer to Rift Valley Fever Virus. Emerg Infect Dis 2018;24(9):1717–9.

10. Tantely LM, Boyer S, Fontenille D. A review of mosquitoes associated with Rift Valley fever virus in Madagascar. Am J Trop Med Hyg 2015;92(4):722–9.

11. Davies FG, Linthicum KJ, James AD. Rainfall and epizootic Rift Valley fever. Bull World Health Organ 1985;63(5):941–3.

12. Gargan TP 2nd, Jupp PG, Novak RJ. Panveld oviposition sites of floodwater Aedes mosquitoes and attempts to detect transovarial transmission of Rift Valley fever virus in South Africa. Med Vet Entomol 1988;2(3):231–6.

13. Bergren NA, Borland EM, Hartman DA, et al. Laboratory demonstration of the vertical transmission of Rift Valley fever virus by Culex tarsalis mosquitoes. PLoS Neglected Trop Dis 2021;15(3):e0009273.

14. Rissmann M, Stoek F, Pickin MJ, et al. Mechanisms of inter-epidemic maintenance of Rift Valley fever phlebovirus. Antivir Res 2020;174:104692.

15. Daubney R, Hudson JR, Garnham PC. Enzootic hepatitis or Rift Valley fever. An undescribed virus disease of sheep cattle and man from East Africa. J Pathol Bacteriol 1931;34(4):545–79.

16. Bird BH, Khristova ML, Rollin PE, et al. Complete genome analysis of 33 ecologically and biologically diverse Rift Valley fever virus strains reveals widespread virus movement and low genetic diversity due to recent common ancestry. J Virol 2007;81(6):2805–16.

17. Bowring CC, Harcourt L. East Africa protectorate. Colonial reports-annual. London: Barclay and Fry; 1914.

18. Gibson S, Noronha LE, Tubbs H, et al. The increasing threat of Rift Valley fever virus globalization: strategic guidance for protection and preparation. J Med Entomol 2023;60(6):1197–213.

19. Lozach PY, Kühbacher A, Meier R, et al. DC-SIGN as a receptor for phleboviruses. Cell Host Microbe 2011;10(1):75–88.

20. Smith DR, Steele KE, Shamblin J, et al. The pathogenesis of Rift Valley fever virus in the mouse model. Virology 2010;407(2):256–67.

21. Schwarz MM, Ganaie SS, Feng A, et al. Lrp1 is essential for lethal Rift Valley fever hepatic disease in mice. Sci Adv 2023;9(28):eadh2264.

22. Gerken KN, Maluni J, Mutuku FM, et al. Exploring potential risk pathways with high risk groups for urban Rift Valley fever virus introduction, transmission, and persistence in two urban centers of Kenya. PLoS Neglected Trop Dis 2023; 17(1):e0010460.

23. de Glanville WA, Allan KJ, Nyarobi JM, et al. An outbreak of Rift Valley fever among peri-urban dairy cattle in northern Tanzania. Trans R Soc Trop Med Hyg 2022;116(11):1082–90.

24. de Glanville WA, Nyarobi JM, Kibona T, et al. Inter-epidemic Rift Valley fever virus infection incidence and risks for zoonotic spillover in northern Tanzania. PLoS Neglected Trop Dis 2022;16(10):e0010871.

25. Coetzer JA. The pathology of Rift Valley fever. II. Lesions occurring in field cases in adult cattle, calves and aborted foetuses. Onderstepoort J Vet Res 1982; 49(1):11–7.

26. Olaleye OD, Tomori O, Fajimi JL, et al. Experimental infection of three Nigerian breeds of sheep with the Zinga strain of the Rift Valley Fever virus. Rev Elev Med Vet Pays Trop 1996;49(1):6–16.

27. Bird BH, Ksiazek TG, Nichol ST, et al. Rift Valley fever virus. J Am Vet Med Assoc 2009;234(7):883–93.

28. Scott GR, Coackley W, Roach RW, et al. Rift Valley fever in camels. J Pathol Bacteriol 1963;86:229–31.

29. Fagbo S, Coetzer JA, Venter EH. Seroprevalence of Rift Valley fever and lumpy skin disease in African buffalo (Syncerus caffer) in the Kruger National Park and Hluhluwe-iMfolozi Park, South Africa. J S Afr Vet Assoc 2014;85(1):e1–7.

30. Antonis AF, Kortekaas J, Kant J, et al. Vertical transmission of Rift Valley fever virus without detectable maternal viremia. Vector Borne Zoonotic Dis 2013;13(8):601–6.

31. Odendaal L, Clift SJ, Fosgate GT, et al. Ovine Fetal and Placental Lesions and Cellular Tropism in Natural Rift Valley Fever Virus Infections. Vet Pathol 2020;57(6):791–806.

32. Anywaine Z, Lule SA, Hansen C, et al. Clinical manifestations of Rift Valley fever in humans: Systematic review and meta-analysis. PLoS Neglected Trop Dis 2022;16(3):e0010233.

33. WHO. Rift Valley Fever Fact Sheet. 2018 cited 2023; Available at: https://www.who.int/news-room/fact-sheets/detail/rift-valley-fever.

34. Yassin W. Clinico-pathological picture in five human cases died with Rift Valley fever. J Egypt Publ Health Assoc 1978;53(3–4):191–3.

35. Swanepoel R, Manning B, Watt JA. Fatal Rift Valley fever of man in Rhodesia. Cent Afr J Med 1979;25(1):1–8.

36. Siam AL, Meegan JM, Gharbawi KF. Rift Valley fever ocular manifestations: observations during the 1977 epidemic in Egypt. Br J Ophthalmol 1980;64(5):366–74.

37. van Velden DJ, Meyer JD, Olivier J, et al. Rift Valley fever affecting humans in South Africa: a clinicopathological study. S Afr Med J 1977;51(24):867–71.

38. Ikegami T, Makino S. The pathogenesis of Rift Valley fever. Viruses 2011;3(5):493–519.

39. Wilson WC, Davis AS, Gaudreault NN, et al. Experimental Infection of Calves by Two Genetically-Distinct Strains of Rift Valley Fever Virus. Viruses 2016;8(5).

40. Odendaal L, Davis AS, Venter EH. Insights into the Pathogenesis of Viral Haemorrhagic Fever Based on Virus Tropism and Tissue Lesions of Natural Rift Valley Fever. Viruses 2021;13(4).

41. Odendaal L, Clift SJ, Fosgate GT, et al. Lesions and Cellular Tropism of Natural Rift Valley Fever Virus Infection in Adult Sheep. Vet Pathol 2019;56(1):61–77.

42. Barski M, Brennan B, Miller OK, et al. Rift Valley fever phlebovirus NSs protein core domain structure suggests molecular basis for nuclear filaments. Elife 2017;6.

43. Petrova V, Kristiansen P, Norheim G, et al. Rift valley fever: diagnostic challenges and investment needs for vaccine development. BMJ Glob Health 2020;5(8).

44. WOAH, Rift Valley Fever, in Manual of Diagnostic Tests and Vaccines for Terrestirial Animal. 2023.

45. Ragan IK, Schuck KN, Upreti D, et al. Rift Valley Fever Viral RNA Detection by In Situ Hybridization in Formalin-Fixed, Paraffin-Embedded Tissues. Vector Borne Zoonotic Dis 2019;19(7):553–6.

46. Smithburn KC. Rift Valley fever; the neurotropic adaptation of the virus and the experimental use of this modified virus as a vaccine. Br J Exp Pathol 1949;30(1):1–16.

47. Anthony T, van Schalkwyk A, Romito M, et al. Vaccination with Rift Valley fever virus live attenuated vaccine strain Smithburn caused meningoencephalitis in alpacas. J Vet Diagn Invest 2021;33(4):777–81.
48. Botros B, Omar A, Elian K, et al. Adverse response of non-indigenous cattle of European breeds to live attenuated Smithburn Rift Valley fever vaccine. J Med Virol 2006;78(6):787–91.
49. Faburay B, LaBeaud AD, McVey DS, et al. Current Status of Rift Valley Fever Vaccine Development. Vaccines (Basel) 2017;5(3).
50. Muller R, Saluzzo JF, Lopez N, et al. Characterization of clone 13, a naturally attenuated avirulent isolate of Rift Valley fever virus, which is altered in the small segment. Am J Trop Med Hyg 1995;53(4):405–11.
51. Makoschey B, van Kilsdonk E, Hubers WR, et al. Rift Valley Fever Vaccine Virus Clone 13 Is Able to Cross the Ovine Placental Barrier Associated with Foetal Infections, Malformations, and Stillbirths. PLoS Neglected Trop Dis 2016;10(3): e0004550.
52. Ikegami T. Rift Valley fever vaccines: an overview of the safety and efficacy of the live-attenuated MP-12 vaccine candidate. Expert Rev Vaccines 2017;16(6): 601–11.
53. Hunter P, Erasmus BJ, Vorster JH. Teratogenicity of a mutagenised Rift Valley fever virus (MVP 12) in sheep. Onderstepoort J Vet Res 2002;69(1):95–8.
54. Jenkin D, Wright D, Folegatti PM, et al. Safety and immunogenicity of a ChAdOx1 vaccine against Rift Valley fever in UK adults: an open-label, non-randomised, first-in-human phase 1 clinical trial. Lancet Infect Dis 2023;23(8):956–64.
55. Wichgers Schreur PJ, Oymans J, Kant J, et al. A single vaccination with four-segmented rift valley fever virus prevents vertical transmission of the wild-type virus in pregnant ewes. NPJ Vaccines 2021;6(1):8.
56. Kitandwe PK, McKay PF, Kaleebu P, et al. An Overview of Rift Valley Fever Vaccine Development Strategies. Vaccines (Basel) 2022;10(11).

Transboundary Tick and Tick-Borne Pathogen Threats to Cattle

Pete D. Teel, BS, MS, PhD[a],*, Thomas Hairgrove, BS, DVM, PhD[b]

KEYWORDS

- Ticks • Tick-borne pathogens • Disease • Surveillance • Diagnosis
- Prompt intervention

KEY POINTS

- Incursions of exotic ticks and tick-borne pathogens are constant transboundary risks for the US cattle industries.
- Vigilance, surveillance, education, and communication are essential national needs from all animal industry and professional partners to prevent, detect, and respond to exotic tick incursions.
- Integrated approaches are required to detect and eliminate tick incursions before they spread, and certainly if they spread beyond containment.
- Integrated approaches to tick suppression can reduce the risk of pathogen transmission.
- Differential diagnostic challenges exist where clinical signs of exotic tick-borne diseases mimic those of bovine anaplasmosis.

INTRODUCTION

Global trade of livestock and wildlife is of great concern to national and international animal industries and agencies involved in animal and human health.[1,2] This is particularly true where potential risks for transport and dispersal of ticks and tick-borne pathogens are possible[3,4] and where introductions of exotic wildlife are likely to expand tick host range.[5] The focus of this article is (1) to draw attention specifically to the transboundary nature, risks, and challenges associated with exotic ticks and tick-borne pathogens of cattle, (2) to highlight the importance of constant vigilance, education, communication, surveillance, response, and enforcement at global to local levels, and (3) to recommend routine practices for small and large animal veterinary practitioners, technicians, producers, extension specialists, and others involved in

[a] Department of Entomology, Texas A&M AgriLife Research, Room 412 Heep Center, 370 Olsen Boulevard, College Station, TX 77843-2475, USA; [b] Department of Animal Science, Texas A&M AgriLife Extension, 241 Kleberg Building, 474 Olsen Boulevard, College Station, TX 77843, USA
* Corresponding author.
E-mail address: Pete.Teel@ag.tamu.edu

Vet Clin Food Anim 40 (2024) 305–316
https://doi.org/10.1016/j.cvfa.2024.01.006
0749-0720/24/© 2024 Elsevier Inc. All rights reserved.

vetfood.theclinics.com

beef and dairy cattle industries as part of the *first line of defense* vigilance, education, communication, surveillance, and response (**Fig. 1**).

The primary concept of national and international boundaries is to establish sovereignty for control of commerce and related activities under law. The US animal industries and animal health associations and agencies provide leadership in developing legislation, policy, and protocols for biosecurity (see **Fig. 1**) regarding lawful global cattle trade, and for surveillance, response, and enforcement against transboundary tick and tick-borne pathogen threats. Transboundary threats for introductions can occur through several pathways and are made complicated by wide host ranges of

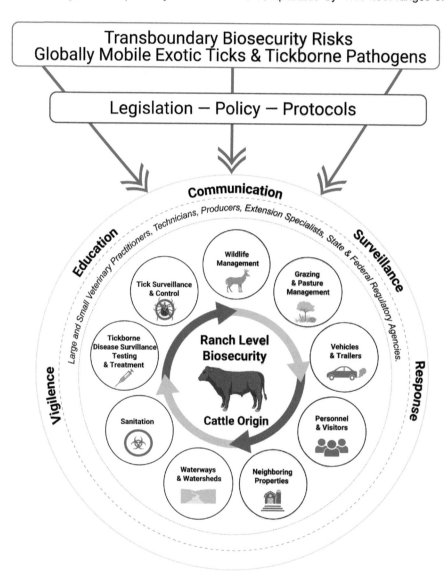

Fig. 1. Summary assessment of threats and control points for transboundary biosecurity risks associated with exotic ticks and tick-borne pathogens from national to local boundary levels.

exotic tick species. Increasing globalization with advances in technologies, transportation, communication, and international cooperation have increased pathways of trade and transport of domestic, companion, and wild animals through legal and illegal channels.[6] Regulations for tick inspection, treatment, and pathogen testing of animals in legal trade channels vary by species and oversight agency, but not all animals are subject to regulation. Higher risks are associated with illegal animal trade channels where oversight, inspection, testing, and treatment are absent. Yet another potential transboundary pathway is through tick-infested birds in migratory flyways that can disperse blood-fed ticks into the United States after having flown considerable distances.[7,8]

Records of exotic ticks collected in the United States in the latter half of the twentieth century illustrate the scope of risks associated with imported livestock and wildlife, as well as animal hides, and in some cases on plant materials.[9,10] With respect to transport of ticks on plant materials, it should be remembered that many tick species seek their next host by climbing vegetation to await the opportunity of their next host blood-meal, and the greatest portion of tick life histories is spent in off-host environments. Ninety-five tick species exotic to the United States were assigned to 9 genera of the family Ixodidae (hard ticks).[9,10] Ticks with known origins included Central and South America, Africa, Middle East, Asia, Europe, and Caribbean, whereas the origin of most were unknown. Hosts from which ticks were collected included diverse taxa of birds, reptiles, and mammals. Most concerning is that collections included vectors of exotic pathogens of bovine diseases (including *Anaplasma, Babesia, Ehrlichia, Theileria*, Crimean-Congo Hemorrhagic Fever Virus, louping-ill virus, and lumpy skin disease virus), and these ticks were collected from diverse non-bovine hosts. Global connections illustrate the need for broad-based awareness and persistent actions to detect incursions of ticks and associated risks of tick-borne pathogens.

Incursions of ticks across boundaries can lead to infestations of animals and premises that can result in outbreaks across many premises and landscapes. Whether an infestation becomes established, and if so, how rapidly it grows and spreads depends on many factors including the following.

- Type of tick biology and reproduction
- Host range and host spread (home range expansion or human-assisted expansion) by tick stage (larva, nymph, adult)
- Habitat and seasonal ecology
- Climatic range
- Among other factors

Preventing incursions of ticks and tick-borne pathogens across boundaries is an essential function of regulatory control, but this line of defense cannot be comprehensive against illegal incursions and bird flyway pathways. Thus, the line of defense must be extended to all who work in animal health and production, including veterinary practitioners, technicians, livestock producers, extension specialists, and state and federal regulatory personnel (see **Fig. 1**). Early detection is essential to early elimination.

DISCUSSION

There are 3 examples of transboundary invasions of different tick and tick-borne disease pathogens of bovines that highlight associated challenges, risks, and realities in the following sections. The examples not only provide comparisons of consequences from different tick species and pathogens, but of circumstances that present current and future challenges and risks unique to each example. The examples underscore recommendations for local, national, and international vigilance and surveillance actions and practices for consistent collection and identification of ticks, the testing and treatment for tick-borne pathogens of cattle, awareness of risks to other animals and humans, and early intervention for exotic tick elimination.

Transboundary Invasion: Asian Long-Horned Tick and Theileria orientalis Ikeda

The Asian long-horned tick, *Haemaphysalis longicornis*, was discovered infesting sheep in New Jersey in 2017. Surveillance by local, state, and federal sources have found *H longicornis* in 19 states as of October 2023, and its range expansion is expected to continue based on climate matching and habitat suitability modeling.[11,12] Retrospective assessments of tick collections suggest that *H longicornis* may have been present since 2010. Genetic evaluation of the global *Cox I* gene haplotype diversity in *H longicornis* indicates that the US tick strain is associated with 3 haplotypes, suggesting comparatively minimal genetic diversity.[13] *H longicornis* is a 3-host tick with a wide host range, wide climatic range and, depending on the strain, can reproduce sexually or asexually. The *H longicornis* strain in the United States is asexual parthenogenic, meaning that reproduction is completed without males and having the capacity to build large populations rapidly.[14] Cattle are a dominant host, subject to high levels of infestation. Reduction of *H longicornis* on infested cow–calf farms in east Tennessee was most successful through an integrated program of tick habitat alteration by shredding overgrown grasses and weeds, strategic acaricide applications to cattle, and maintenance of closed herds.[15]

Cattle presenting with a febrile illness on a Virginia farm on which there was an *H longicornis* infestation were found positive for *Theileria orientalis* Ikeda strain.[16] Subsequently, laboratory transmission of a *T orientalis* Ikeda isolate from the Virginia site by the US strain of *H longicornis* was confirmed.[17] Cattle in multiple states known to have *H longicornis* infestations have now been diagnosed with *T orientalis* Ikeda infections,[18] and it is likely that *T orientalis* Ikeda will follow the expected geographic expansion of *H longicornis*.

T orientalis Ikeda is a tick-borne protozoan parasite that has negatively impacted the cattle industries in Japan, Australia, and New Zealand, especially after introducing naïve or severely stressed cattle into endemic areas.[19] European breeds are more susceptible to disease than Zebu breeds. *H longicornis* ticks are the primary vectors of the pathogen; however, vertical transmission from pregnant cows to their calves and mechanical transmission by biting tabanid flies, sucking lice, and contaminated vaccination needles and surgical instruments potentially transfer infected erythrocytes. Affected animals demonstrate anemia, high fever, lacrimation, nasal discharge, swollen lymph nodes, and hemoglobinuria. Australia reported significant abortions, deaths, and declines in milk production in beef and dairy cattle. Postmortem lesions include abomasal ulcers, splenomegaly, and massive pulmonary edema.

In September 2017, a beef cattle herd in Virginia developed anemia, and *Anaplasma marginale* was suspected. Blood samples tested by polymerase chain reaction (PCR) failed to confirm *A marginale,* but blood smears revealed pleomorphic piroplasms.[16] This index case identified *T orientalis* Ikeda, genotype 2, not previously identified in the United States as the primary pathogen.[17] Other genotypes of *T orientalis* are present in the United States, but outbreaks are uncommon and related to the clinically benign Buffeli genotype.[17] In the absence of current approved treatments for clinical *T orientalis* Ikeda, integrated approaches that minimize the movement of naïve cattle into endemic areas and apply integrated tick management applications on infested properties for tick suppression can reduce transmission risk.[14,15,20]

Transboundary Invasion: Cattle Fever Ticks: Babesia bigemina and B Bovis

Rhipicephalus (Boophilus) annulatus and *R (B) microplus*, collectively known as cattle fever ticks (CFTs), and bovine babesiosis, also known as Texas cattle fever among other names, caused by the apicomplexan protozoa, *Babesia bigemina,* and *B bovis*, were once prevalent across 13 southern states and southern California.[21] The combined effects of tick parasitism and babesiosis on cattle and cattle production enterprises in the nineteenth century were significant, both economically and in being technically detrimental to animal agriculture development in the twentieth century.[22] CFTs were the responsible source for *Babesia* transmission from infected to noninfected cattle leading to disease. Practices such as pasture rotation to fallowed ground and pasture vacation allowed ticks dropping from infested cattle to die in an inhospitable habitat, or die in the absence of a subsequent host, respectfully, and chemical-based techniques for treatment of CFT-infested cattle, brought about the successful elimination of babesiosis through a state-federal Cattle Fever Tick Eradication Program[22] initiated in 1906. Although CFT eradication was declared complete in 1943, CFT incursions into the Texas border region on infested livestock from Mexico continued prompting the establishment of a narrow quarantine zone along the Rio Grande.[23] Today, the US Department of Agriculture (USDA) Animal and Plant Health Inspection Service (APHIS) Veterinary Services (VS) Tick Force provides tick surveillance, livestock apprehension, treatment, and enforcement of CFT eradication in the buffer zone, whereas the Texas Animal Health Commission provides state-wide passive surveillance of ticks, as well as response to CFT infestations that occur beyond the buffer zone.

Transboundary challenges currently affect the Cattle Fever Tick Eradication Program. Acaricide resistance emerged among CFT populations in Mexico, and resistant ticks are among those making their way across the Rio Grande into Texas.[24] The reestablishment of white-tailed deer and introductions of exotic wildlife ungulates, including nilgai antelope, *Boselaphus tragocamelus* (Bovidae), an original host for *R (B) microplus* from India, have compromised the application of pasture vacation as an eradication technique and expanded the scope of epidemiology and treatment protocols for CFT infestations.[5,25] Changes in land-use, property ownership transfers with changes in premise sizes, periodic droughts, and economic pressures all contribute to changes along the border quarantine zone and south Texas with impacts on operational activities of the Cattle Fever Tick Eradication Program.[21,26]

These challenges underscore the need for integrated approaches to CFT eradication with broad systematic active surveillance and novel technological developments for detection and anti-CFT treatments across multiple host species.[21,27] Cattle fever tick incursions and outbreaks inside Texas have occurred in recent years. Epidemiologic trace outs of livestock from infestation sites in the 12-month period before discovery demonstrate mobility of animals and potential risk of CFT dispersal to counties across Texas and to many states beyond Texas.

Transboundary challenges of tick-borne disease can also exist with cattle legally imported or that stray into Texas from Mexico. Both CFT species and *Babesia* pathogens remain endemic in Mexico. It is estimated that 52% of the national Mexican territory is infested with *R (B) annulatus* and/or *R (B) microplus* and that approximately 75% of Mexican cattle are subject to babesia infection.[28] Between 2018 and 2021, from 1.1 to 1.4 million head of Mexican cattle were legally imported annually into the United States.[29] Many of these imported cattle are considered light-weight stockers and are placed on wheat or grass pastures throughout the country for growth and maturity. Imported cattle are inspected and certified CFT-free, but they may be infected with either *B bigemina* or *B bovis* or another tick-borne pathogen such as *A marginale* acknowledged to be endemic in Mexico.[30] A recent survey of stray Mexican cattle from 8 Texas border counties found 58.5% of 135 samples were positive for one or more of these 3 pathogens by PCR testing, and 15% of samples were indicated to be coinfections.[31] *Rhipicephalus (B) microplus* and *R (B) annulatus* are among ixodid tick species known to vector *A marginale* globally.[32] Cattle coming into the United States with coinfections may present practitioners with diagnostic challenges arising from shared clinical signs, inconclusive or confusing diagnostic test results, and unknown travel/owner histories.

Transboundary Dilemma: A marginale: A Confounding Factor for Diagnosing Transboundary Bovine Tick-Borne Pathogens

Similarities in clinical manifestations of transboundary bovine diseases associated with *T orientalis*, *B bigemina*, and *B bovis* occurring in US endemic areas of bovine anaplasmosis, and particularly in the absence of key tick species [*H longicornis*, *R (B) annulatus* or *R (B) microplus*] can result in challenging diagnoses for practitioners.

A marginale, an obligate intracellular gram-negative rickettsial bacterium, causes bovine anaplasmosis. The disease is not considered a transboundary disease, but is considered a "monitored disease" by the USDA defined as an endemic disease assessed by monthly reporting by the state animal health officials and APHIS VS to monitor changes over time. It is considered endemic in most of the United States, Mexico, and Central and South America. Globally, *A marginale* is the most prevalent tick-borne infection, negatively affecting livestock production in tropical and subtropical regions.[33] The disease is found on all 6 continents, is diagnosed in most states in the United States, and is endemic in tropical and subtropical areas of the world. *A marginale* is transmitted biologically by some 20 species of ticks, mechanically transmitted by biting flies, and blood-contaminated instruments and transmitted vertically from an infected dam to her fetus.[32] *A marginale* invades and replicates in ruminant erythrocytes and in the midgut and salivary glands of certain ticks, making them efficient biological vectors. The infected erythrocytes of cattle become phagocytized by the reticuloendothelial system, which causes the production of anti-erythrocyte antibodies, the release of acute-phase inflammatory agents, and accompanying anemia and fever.[19] Cattle that survive acute infection remain persistently infected for life but do not show clinical disease unless immunosuppressed by factors such as malnutrition, stress, or extreme pathogen load. Persistent infection allows animals to maintain immunity and resistance to clinical disease through "sequential antigenic variation." As the number of circulating bacteria increases, they trigger a host's antibody response, diminishing infected circulating bacteria. As the bacteria decline, their major surface proteins alter, allowing them to evade the host's immune response until the changes are recognized, and the immune system partially compromises the pathogen again. This cycle results in a bimonthly variation in the concentration of infected erythrocytes varying from 10^3 to 10^5 infected cells/mL of blood, lower than the 10^9 infected cells/mL seen in acute infection.[19]

Animals infected before 6 months of age seldom exhibit clinical disease, and cattle infected before 20 months may show clinical signs but rarely die. Mortality rates of 29% to 49% are not uncommon in naïve adult cattle experiencing acute anaplasmosis. Acute infection results in fever (103 °F–106 °F) that subsides within a day, dropping to normal or subnormal. There is muzzle dryness, suppression of rumen activity, and often constipation.[33] Cattle can become aggressive, and cows abort due to cerebral hypoxia associated with severe anemia. Mature cattle recovering from acute anaplasmosis are reservoirs for transmission of *A marginale* to naïve cattle. Definitive diagnosis of acute *A marginale* requires identifying the organism and a significantly low hematocrit.

Differential diagnoses include babesiosis, bacillary hemoglobinuria, leptospirosis, and other liver conditions producing icterus.[33] Following the introductions of *H longicornis* and *T orientalis* Ikeda, it was recognized that clinical theileriosis can mimic bovine anaplasmosis.[34] The occurrence of cattle in Virginia with coinfections of *T orientalis* Ikeda and *A marginale* underscored the need for reliable differential diagnostic tests such as a duplex reverse transcription polymerase chain reaction (rtPCR) assay.[34] Although *H longicornis* is not a recognized vector of *A marginale*,[35] other ticks in the area, including *Dermacentor variabilis*,[36] are known vectors of *A marginale*,[32,37] indicating the presence of multiple biological vector–pathogen systems. The expected spread of *H longicornis* will undoubtedly include other areas endemic for bovine anaplasmosis, and differential diagnoses will become essential.

Treatment for acute bovine anaplasmosis centers on the parenteral use of injectable oxytetracycline. Continuous feeding of chlortetracycline (CTC) can control active infection caused by *A marginale*.[32] Therefore, continuous feeding of CTC to cattle for anaplasmosis control during the vector season is considered standard practice. Currently, there are no effective and approved treatments for *T orientalis* Ikeda in the United States.

The dilemma of coinfections of tick-borne pathogens is not uncommon. In 2017, a 450-cow dairy in Panama, Central America was experiencing deaths from acute *A marginale* with 2 shipments of 20 month old heifers imported from the United States. The dairy was located in an endemic area for *R (B) microplus* ticks. In molecular testing of 108 animals, 100% were PCR positive for *A marginale,* and 82% of animals were concurrently infected with *Babesia* (Hairgrove, unpublished data, 2017). When cattle become dually infected with a transboundary disease with clinical signs similar to bovine anaplasmosis, often the disease investigation ceases especially in areas where anaplasmosis is endemic, possibly overlooking the introduction of a significant transboundary disease.

Transboundary Invasion: Tropical Bont Tick and Ehrlichia ruminantium

Heartwater is an African disease of domestic and wild ruminants, caused by *Ehrlichia ruminantium*, and vectored by as many as 13 *Amblyomma* tick species from that continent, particularly *A variegatum* and *A hebraeum*.[38] It has never been found in the United States. The disease is highly fatal in naïve cattle, with clinical cases presenting with fever, nervous disorders, hydropericardia, and gastroenteritis. The tropical bont tick, *A variegatum*, is of particular interest to the United States because of its presence in the Caribbean and proximity to the mainland. It had been resident on the southern leeward islands of Marie Galante and Guadeloupe for more than a century; however in the 1970s, it began spreading and ultimately infested 18 islands by the late 1980s.[7] *E ruminantium* was detected on 3 islands (Marie Galant, Guadeloupe, and Antigua).

Cattle egrets, *Bubulcus ibis*, expanded into the Caribbean during the decades between 1950 and 1970,[39] becoming a common sight among grazing cattle, sheep, and goats. Surveys of cattle egrets on the islands discovered the birds were infested with larvae and to a lesser extent nymphs of *A variegatum,* and proportions of marked birds from three islands were subsequently reported on 14 Caribbean islands and the Florida Keys,[40] illustrating the potential role of cattle egret inter-island migration on Caribbean spread and risk to the US Gulf Coast.

An international effort to eradicate *A variegatum* from the Caribbean was undertaken in 1994[41] and ended in 2008 leaving resident tick populations that survived the eradication campaign.[42] The island of St. Croix, US Virgin Islands, has been repeatedly reinfested with *A variegatum* following US eradication.[43] Two native *Amblyomma* species, the Gulf Coast tick, *A maculatum*, and the cayenne tick, *A cajennense* (now recognized as *A mixtum*), were determined to be putative vectors of *E ruminantium*, increasing concerns posed by *A variegatum* and heartwater potentially entering the United States.[44] Surveillance and early detection of *Amblyomma variegatum* along the Gulf Coast and Atlantic states is critical to any intervention to contain spread of ticks and risk of heartwater cases.

The presence of *A variegatum* in tropical climates of Africa has been connected to increased occurrence of severe dermatophilosis in cattle, sheep, and goats,[45] and this association has also been made in the Caribbean islands of Antigua[46] and St. Lucia.[47] Dermatophilosis, or cutaneous streptothricosis, is caused by *Dermatophilosis congolensis*, actinomycete bacteria that produces filamentous hyphae in epidermal scabs and ultimately produces ovoid zoospores.[45] Transstadial transmission of *D congolensis* (larvae to nymphs; nymphs to adults) in *A variegatum* was negative in sheep.[48] However, studies with blood-feeding *A variegatum* suggest that systemic effects of adult tick feeding stimulate clinical manifestations of dermatophilosis in subclinical carrier animals through immunologic means.[48,49] Numerous authors have noted that tick suppression of *A variegatum* brings about declines in clinical dermatophilosis. In the absence of active tick surveillance programs along the southern Gulf Coast of the United States, an unusual increase in cases of dermatophilosis should be cause for close animal inspection for ticks and submission of samples for identification.

SUMMARY

Threats to the health and well-being of US cattle from exotic ticks and tick-borne pathogens are ever present and growing due to globalization of animal trade channels. Although policies and procedures are in place to detect and prevent introductions, ticks still cross US boundaries, and often as not, it is a client or practitioner who makes critical first discoveries. Vigilance, education, communication, surveillance, and response have been illustrated as *the first line of defense*, and participants include veterinary practitioners, technicians, producers, extension specialists, and others involved in beef and dairy cattle industries (see **Fig. 1**).

CLINICS CARE POINTS

- Transboundary movement of ticks and tick-borne pathogens is a priority. In addition, several native tick species are undergoing range expansion in the United States facilitated by movement of hosts, host range expansion, and changing climate and weather patterns. Integrate routine practices for animal inspections into your operational activities and clinical practices. Stay abreast of latest findings on clinical signs and diagnostics for tick-borne pathogens.

- Recognize that whenever animals move, ticks and tick-borne pathogens are also likely on the move. This is true across national and international boundaries as well as state boundaries and the boundaries of personal property/operation. Exercising biosecurity precautions at all boundaries can improve early detection and intervention and slow expansion.

- Economic changes and drought recovery are 2 examples that drive cattle sales and herd rebuilding cycles. When rebuilding or expanding herds, clients should learn about the source area and history of the cattle to be purchased. To prevent introducing something unwanted, inspect and identify ticks encountered, treat cattle to remove ticks, and quarantine new animals for observation and conduct appropriate diagnostic testing before mixing them into the resident herd. Avoid risks of moving naïve animals from non-endemic to endemic disease areas.

- Inspection of cattle for ticks is optimally conducted when animals are restrained in a chute or pressed in an alley. Primary body areas of tick attachment are head (around eyes, ears, and nose), leg auxiliaries, belly, udder/scrotum, perineum, and tailhead. Animals with heavy infestations may have ticks on their sides, flanks, and topline. Ticks should be removed by clasping near where the head is imbedded in the skin and slowly pulling away from the body surface without twisting or jerking. This is the optimal method to ensure that the head portion of the tick body is removed. The tick head contains several structures important to accurate/complete identification. Ticks should be placed in a clean container with isopropyl alcohol or ethanol as preservative and labeled with date, location, host, and collector name. Specimens should be submitted for identification to state or federal animal health agencies and laboratories, to land grant universities or academic institutions, or public health organizations with expertise in tick identification.

- Incorporate integrated tick management to suppress ticks and diminish the impacts of heavy tick burden on animal growth and performance as well as the risks of pathogen transmission. Integrated tick management includes tick surveillance and combinations of control methods suitable to location-specific circumstances. Control methods can be directed at managing off-host tick habitat through herbicides, mowing/shredding, or prescribed-burns, and managing on-host tick infestation with applications of approved acaricides at labeled rates. Integrated tick management also applies to control of animals coming into the herd so as not to introduce ticks or tick-borne pathogens.

- Routinely update awareness of changing dynamics in animal trade and recent findings concerning ticks and tick-borne pathogens of livestock, companion animals, wildlife, and humans. Those working in animal health and production are occupationally exposed to ticks and tick-borne pathogens, so they should learn to recognize common symptoms and exposure points. Canine and equine working animals can also be exposed, and care should be taken to include them in surveillance and treatment as needed. Proper tick removal and submission for pathogen testing can be helpful.

- Veterinarians should work with their cattle clients to develop a biosecurity program based on their operation's risks for ticks and tick-borne disease pathogens.

ACKNOWLEDGMENTS

The authors are grateful for the assistance of Dr Taylor Donaldson and Dr Samantha Hays, Texas A&M Agrilife Research, for article review and graphic assistance.

DISCLOSURE

The authors have no commercial or financial conflict of interest in the content of this article.

REFERENCES

1. Clemmons EA, Alfson KJ, Dutton JW III. Transboundary animal diseases, an overview of 17 diseases with potential for global spread and serious consequences. Animals 2021;11:2039.
2. World Organization for Animal Health. Animal Diseases. Animal Diseases - WOAH - World Organisation for Animal Health. Accessed October 3, 2023.
3. Tiffin HS, Rajotte EG, Sakamoto JM, et al. Tick control in a connected world: challenges, solutions, and public policy from a United States border perspective. Tropical Medicine and Infectious Disease 2022;7:388.

4. Dantas-Torres F, Chomel BB, Otranto D. Ticks and tick-borne diseases: a one health perspective. Trends Parasitol 2012;28(10):437–46.

5. Sliwa KM, Baumgardt JA, DeYoung RW, et al. Movement ecology of exotic nilgai antelope: a threat to the re-emergence of cattle fever ticks in the southern USA. Ecosphere 2023;14:e4401.

6. Food and Agriculture Organization of the United Nations. GF-TADs Strategy for 2021-2025 Enhancing control of transboundary animal diseases for global health 2021.

7. Barre N, Uilenberg G, Morel PC, et al. Danger of introducing heartwater onto the American mainland: Potential role of indigenous and exotic Amblyomma ticks. Onderstepoort J Vet Res 1987;54:405–17.

8. Scott JD, Durden LA. First record of *Amblyomma rotundatum* tick (Acari: Ixodidae) parasitizing a bird collected in Canada. Syst Appl Acarol 2015;20(2): 155–61.

9. Keirans JE, Durden LA. Invasion: Exotic ticks (Acari: Argasidae, Ixodidae) imported into the United States. A review and new records. J Med Entomol 2001; 38(6):850–61.

10. Burridge MJ, Simmons LA. Exotic ticks introduced into the United States on imported reptiles from 1962 to 2001 and their potential roles in international dissemination of diseases. Vet Parasitol 2003;113:289–320.

11. Raghavan RK, Barker SC, Cobos ME, et al. Potential spatial distribution of the newly introduced long-horned tick, Haemaphysalis longicornis in North America. Sci Rep 2019;9:498. https://doi.org/10.1038/s41598-018-37205-2.

12. Namgyal J, Couloigner I, Lysyk TJ, et al. Comparison of habitat suitability models for *Haemaphysalis longicornis* Newmann in North America to determine its potential geographic range. Int J Environ Res Publ Health 2020;17:8285. https://doi.org/10.3390/ijerph17218285.

13. Egizi A, Bulaga-Seraphin L, Alt E, et al. First glimpse into the origin and spread of the Asian longhorned tick, *Haemaphysalis longicornis*, in the United States. Zoonoses Public Health 2020;67:637–50. https://doi.org/10.1111/zph.12743.

14. Schappach BL, Krell RK, Hornbostel VL, et al. Exotic *Haemaphysalis longicornis* (Acari: Ixodidae) in the United States: Biology, ecology, and strategies for management. J. Integrated Pest Mgmt 2020;11(1):1–11.

15. Butler RA, Trout Fryxell RT. Management of *Haemaphysalis longicornis* (Acari: Ixodidae) on a cow-calf farm in East Tennessee, USA. J Med Entomol 2023;60(6): 1374–9.

16. Oakes VJ, Yabsley MJ, Schwartz D, et al. *Theileria orientalis* Ikeda genotype in cattle, Virginia, USA. Emerg Infect Dis 2019;25(9):1653–9.

17. Dinkel KD, Herndon DR, Noh SM, et al. Isolate of *Theileria orientalis*, Ikeda genotype, is transmitted to cattle by the invasive Asian longhorned tick, *Haemaphysalis longicornis*. Parasites Vectors 2021;14:157.

18. Onzere CK, Hassan A, Herndon DR, et al. *Dermacentor variabilis* does not transtadially transmit the U.S. isolate of *Theileria orientalis* Ikeda: A controlled acquisition and transmission study. Parasitologia 2023;3:284–92.

19. Constable P, Hinchcliff K, Done S, et al. Anaplasmosis due to *A. marginale* and *A. ovis*. Veterinary Medicine: a textbook of diseases of cattle, horses, sheep, pigs, and goats. St. Louis, MO: Elsevier; 2017. p. 769–75.

20. Emery DL. Approaches to integrated parasite management (IPM) for *Theileria orientalis* with an emphasis on immunity. Pathogens 2021;10:1153.

21. Perez de Leon AA, Teel PD, Auclair AN, et al. Integrated strategy for sustainable cattle fever tick eradication in USA is required to mitigate the impact of global change. Front Physiol 2012;3:195.
22. Graham OH, Hourrigan JL. Eradication programs for the arthropod parasites of livestock. J Med Entomol 1977;13(6):629–58.
23. Giles JR, Peterson AT, Busch JD, et al. Invasive potential of cattle fever ticks in the southern United States. Parasites Vectors 2014;7:189.
24. Thomas DB, Klafke G, Busch JD, et al. Tracking the increase of acaricide resistance in an invasive population of cattle fever ticks (Acari: Ixodidae) and implementation of real-time PCR assays to rapidly genotype resistance mutations. Ann Entomol Soc Am 2020;113(4):298–309. https://doi.org/10.1093/aesa/saz053.
25. Busch JD, Stone NE, Nottingham R, et al. Widespread movement of invasive cattle fever ticks (Rhipicephalus microplus) in southern Texas leads to shared local infestations on cattle and deer. Parasites Vectors 2014;7:188.
26. Thompson JM, Delgado AH, Hasel HS, et al. Effects of drought and media-reported violence on cattle fever tick incursions. Frontiers in Vet Sci 2020;7: 373. https://doi.org/10.3389/fvets.2020.00373.
27. Showler AT, Perez de Leon A, Saelao P. Biosurveillance and research needs involving area-wide sampling to enhance integrated cattle fever tick (Ixodida: Ixodidae) eradication. J Med Entomol 2021;58(4):1601–9. https://doi.org/10.1093/jme/tjab051.
28. Esteve-Gasent MD, Rodrigues-Vivas RI, Medina RF, et al. Research on integrated management of cattle fever ticks and bovine babesiosis in the United States and Mexico: Current status and opportunities for binational coordination. Pathogens 2020;9:871.
29. USDA, Economic Research Service, Annual and cumulative year-to-date U.S. livestock and meat trade by country. Published August 2023. Cattle_Yearly-Full.xlsx (live.com). Accessed October 5, 2023.
30. Figueroa JV, Alvarez JA, Ramos JA, et al. Bovine babesiosis and anaplasmosis follow-up on cattle relocated in an endemic area for hemoparasitic diseases. Ann N Y Acad Sci 1998;1–10.
31. Scoles GA, Lohmeyer KH, Ueti MW, et al. Stray Mexico origin cattle captured crossing into Southern Texas carry Babesia bovis and other tick-borne pathogens. Ticks and Tick-borne Diseases 2021;12. https://doi.org/10.1016/j.ttbdis.2021.101708.
32. Aubry P, Geale DW. A review of bovine anaplasmosis. Transboundary and Emerging Diseases 2011;58:1–30. https://doi.org/10.1111/j.1865-1682.2010.01173.x.
33. Palmer GH. Sir Arnold Theiler and the discovery of anaplasmosis: A centennial perspective. Onderstepoort J Vet Res 2009;76:75–9.
34. Oakes VJ, Todd SM, Carbonello AA, et al. Coinfection of cattle in Virginia with Therileris orientalis Ikeda genotype and Anaplasma marginale. J Vet Diagn Invest 2022;14(1):36–41. https://doi.org/10.1177/10406387211057627.
35. Connell ML. Attempted transmission of Anaplasma marginale by Haemaphysalis longicornis. Aust Vet J 1978;54:92–3.
36. Sonenshine DE. Range expansion of tick disease vectors in North America: Implications for spread of tick-borne disease. Int J Environ Res Publ Health 2018; 15:478.
37. Kocan KM, de la Fuente J, Blouin EF, et al. The natural history of Anaplasma marginale. Vet Parasitol 2010;167:95–107.
38. Bram RA, George JE, Reichard RE, et al. Threat of foreign arthropod-borne pathogens to livestock in the United States. J Med Entomol 2002;39(3):405–16.

39. Arendt WJ. Range expansion of the cattle egret (*Bubulcus ibis*) in the greater Caribbean basin. Colon Waterbirds 1988;11(2):252–62.

40. Corn JL, Barre N, Thiebot B, et al. Potential role of cattle egrets, *Bubulcus ibis* (Ciconiformes: Ardeidae), in the dissemination of *Amblyomma variegatum* (Acari: Ixodidae) in the eastern Caribbean. J Med Entomol 1993;30(6):1029–37.

41. Pegram RG, Hansen JW, Wilson DD. Eradication and surveillance of the tropical bont tick in the Caribbean: An international approach. NY Acad Sci 2000;179–85.

42. Ahoussou S, Lancelot R, Sanford B, et al. Analysis of *Amblyomma* surveillance data in the Caribbean: Lessons for future control programmes. Vet Parasitol 2010;167:327–35.

43. Corn JL, Berger P, Mertins JW. Surveys for ectoparasites on wildlife associated with *Amblyomma variegatum* (Acari: Ixodidae)-infested livestock in St. Croix, U.S. Virgin Islands. J Med Entomol 2009;46(6):1483–9.

44. Mahan SM, Peter TF, Simbi BH, et al. Comparison of efficacy of American and African *Amblyomma* ticks as vectors of heartwater (*Cowdria ruminantium*) infection by molecular analyses and transmission trials. J Parasitol 2000;86(1):44–9.

45. Plowright W. Cutaneous streptothricosis of cattle. I. Introduction and epizootiological features in Nigeria. Vet Rec 1956;68:350–5.

46. Morrow AN, Heron ID, Walker AR, et al. *Amblyomma variegatum* ticks and the occurrence of bovine streptothricosis in Antigua. J Vet Med 1989;36:241–9.

47. Morrow AN, Compton EAE. The occurrence of streptothricosis and its association with *Amblyomma variegatum* ticks in St. Lucia. J Vet Med 1991;38:635–8.

48. Martinez D, Barre N, Mari B, et al. Tick Vector Biology: Studies of the role of Amblyomma variegatum in the transmission of Dermatophilosis congolensis. Berlin, Heidelberg: Springer; 1992. https://doi.org/10.1007/978-3-642-76643-5_6.

49. Walker AR, Lloyd CM. Experiments on the relationship between feeding of the tick *Amblyomma variegatum* (Acari: Ixodidae) and dermatophilosis skin disease in sheep. J Med Entomol 1993;30(1):136–43.

Reemerging/Notifiable Diseases to Watch

Sherrilyn H. Wainwright, DVM, MPH[a],*,
Cristina W. Cunha, DVM, MS, PhD[b], Brett Webb, DVM, PhD, DACVP[c],
Bethany McGregor, MS, PhD[d], Barbara Drolet, MS, PhD[d],
John B. Welch, PhD[e]

KEYWORDS

- Gammaherpesvirus • OvHV-2 • SA-MCF • Bluetongue virus • Orbivirus
- New world screwworm • *Cochliomyia hominivorax*

KEY POINTS

- New World screwworm (NWS) is a devastating obligate parasite of warm-blooded animals.
- NWS can negatively affect livestock production, health of companion animals, wildlife populations, and human health. Untreated wounds can lead to the death of the host.
- The concern is the possibility of reintroduction into the United States or other NWS-free areas, most commonly by the transport of NWS-infested animals.
- Screwworm myiasis reporting is mandatory to State Animal Health Officials (SAHO) or the United States Department of Agriculture, Animal and Plant Health Inspection Service (USDA-APHIS).
- Samples should be sent for confirmation to the USDA-APHIS-Veterinary Services, National Veterinary Services Laboratories in Ames, Iowa.

INTRODUCTION

Reemerging and notifiable diseases of cattle and bison continue to pose potential risks to their health and lives, affecting production and the livelihoods of producers. It is essential to understand the clinical presentation of these diseases to watch for possible incursions and infections and to immediately report your suspicions to your State and Federal Animal Health Officials. Malignant catarrhal fever (MCF),

[a] United States Department of Agriculture, Animal and Plant Health Inspection Service, Veterinary Services, 2150 Centre Avenue, Building B, Fort Collins, CO 80526, USA; [b] United States Department of Agriculture, Agricultural Research Service, Animal Disease Research Unit, 3003 ADBF, WSU, Pullman, WA 99164-6630, USA; [c] North Dakota State University, Veterinary Diagnostic Laboratory, 4035 19th Avenue North, Fargo, ND 58102, USA; [d] Agricultural Research Service, United States Department of Agriculture, 1515 College Avenue, Manhattan, KS 66502, USA; [e] United States Department of Agriculture, Animal Plant Health Inspection Service, International Services, Action Programs, 2881 F&B Road, College Station, TX 77845, USA
* Corresponding author.
E-mail address: sherrilyn.h.wainwright@usda.gov

Vet Clin Food Anim 40 (2024) 317–335
https://doi.org/10.1016/j.cvfa.2024.01.007
0749-0720/24/Published by Elsevier Inc.

bluetongue virus, and New World screwworm (NWS), 3 of these reemerging and noti-fiable diseases of cattle and bison, are presented in this article for increased aware-ness to consider as differentials if examinations present suggestive clinical signs. Immediate notification of your State and Federal Officials is essential for appropriate confirmation, investigation, and response to prevent further spread of these poten-tially serious diseases causing harm to animals, production, livelihoods, and, with NWS, public health.

MALIGNANT CATARRHAL FEVER
Malignant Catarrhal Fever Viruses and Their Host Species

Malignant Catarrhal Fever (MCF) is an often fatal disease of many ungulate species caused by a group of gammaherpesviruses in the genus Macavirus, referred to as MCF viruses.[1] According to previous reports, the viruses causing MCF are closely related genetically and present a unique epitope that differentiates them from other lymphotropic Macaviruses.[2] At least 10 MCF viruses have been identified so far; 7 of them are known to cause disease whereas no clinically susceptible species have been identified for the other 3.[3]

Each MCF virus has coevolved with a particular animal species. Consequently, this resulted in adaptation of that species to the virus, and upon infection, these animals usually do not develop the disease but remain as asymptomatic carriers and serve as virus reservoirs. Infectious viral particles are shed sporadically from carrier hosts and can infect nonadapted animals susceptible to developing MCF. In this scenario, it is important to keep in mind that MCF can emerge anywhere carrier and clinically susceptible hosts are kept in proximity to one another.

The vast majority of MCF cases in North America are caused by ovine herpesvirus-2 (OvHV-2), which exists as a common subclinical infection in sheep and causes sheep-associated MCF (SA-MCF) in several ungulates, including bison, cattle, deer, and pigs. Limited information exists about the susceptibility of these animal species to other MCF viruses. The list of known MCF viruses and their adapted and non-adapted hosts reviewed by Li and colleagues can be used as a reference.[3]

Sheep-Associated Malignant Catarrhal Fever Epidemiology

Major risk factors that influence the risk of SA-MCF in cattle and bison and are impor-tant for species management and disease control are illustrated in **Fig. 1**.

- *OvHV-2 is carried by domestic sheep as a lifelong subclinical infection.* Lambs are usually not infected until 2 to 3 months of age but depending on the level of expo-sure, most animals are infected within a year.[4] In the United States, the preva-lence in adult sheep can be greater than 90%.[5,6] Lambs can be raised free of OvHV-2 if separated from infected sheep at an early age prior to infection and are maintained under surveillance with repeated testing to ensure the virus-free status.[4,7] Multispecies operations and zoos have been using this strategy to successfully produce OvHV-2-free sheep as a method to control SA-MCF.[8,9]
- *OvHV-2 is shed into the environment by infected sheep, mostly via nasal secre-tions.*[10] Overall, low amounts of virus can be consistently detected in the nasal secretions and blood of infected animals; however, occurrence of shedding ep-isodes, where large amounts of infectious virus particles are released from nasal secretions, is unpredictable and usually short-lived, lasting less than 24 hours. Lambs aged between 6 and 9 months shed the virus more frequently and inten-sively than adults.[10]

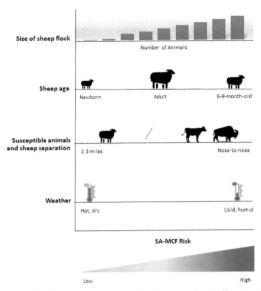

Fig. 1. Major factors that influence the risk of SA-MCF in clinically susceptible species.

- *MCF viruses are not transmitted from clinically affected hosts.* Animals clinically affected with MCF are considered dead-end hosts, do not shed infectious virus, and are not capable of infecting herdmates.[11,12]
- *SA-MCF can occur year-round.* In North America, SA-MCF cases tend to occur in the late fall and winter, when weather conditions and the increased population of adolescent lambs in the pastures and feedlots favor increased exposure to OvHV-2.[10,13]
- *Both adapted and nonadapted species acquire the virus mostly through inhalation.* OvHV-2 is more efficiently transmitted when animals are in close contact. The exact physical distance that prevents transmission is difficult to determine because it is dependent on the susceptible species at risk, the number and age of the sheep, and environmental factors. However, a clear inverse relationship between the number of cases and distance to sheep has been documented in an MCF outbreak in bison, in which transmission still occurred when animals were separated by more than 3 miles.[14] Fomites, including virus-laden secretions and water, may also serve as possible sources of infectious virus but transmission efficiency is expected to be low.
- *MCF viruses are relatively unstable in the environment.* Studies with alcelaphine herpesvirus-1 (AlHV-1), an MCF virus carried by wildebeest, showed that the virus becomes nonviable within 48 hours under hot, dry weather conditions but can be infectious for at least 13 days in humid environments under mild temperatures.[15,16] There are no experimental data for OvHV-2 because its infectivity cannot be confirmed in vitro due to the lack of a cell culture system to propagate the virus; however, its stability is expected to be comparable to other MCF viruses. Common commercially available disinfectants used as recommended by the manufacturer can inactivate MCF viruses.
- *Infection of cattle and bison with OvHV-2 can result in SA-MCF.* Although both species are susceptible to the disease, cattle are relatively more resistant than bison, requiring approximately 1000 times more virus to induce disease.[17,18]

Clinical Manifestation

- *The clinical signs of SA-MCF are similar in cattle and bison with the clinical course varying from peracute to chronic disease with recrudescence.*[19,20] Although cattle display the full spectrum of disease chronicity, bison typically present with the acute or peracute form. Subclinical cases do occur and appear to be more common in cattle than in bison.[19,20]

In both species, the incubation period varies widely (21–270 days) and appears to depend primarily on infectious dose, although other host factors are likely involved.[18,21,22] The clinical course of disease is typically less than 1 week and often 1 to 3 days.[23,24] In the peracute form, animals are often found dead without preceding clinical signs.[21]

Early symptoms are nonspecific and characterized by lethargy, reduced feed intake, high fever (104°F–108°F), and isolation from the herd. Although symptoms of the head and eye seem to predominate,[25] animals can develop any constellation of the following clinical signs: ocular and nasal discharge, corneal edema beginning at the limbus, uveitis, lymphadenomegaly, dermatitis, dyspnea, excessive salivation, oral and nasal planum erosions, corneal edema, hematuria, hematochezia, and neurologic symptoms, such as weakness, ataxia, nystagmus, head pressing, paralysis, and convulsions.[3,26]

- *Although mortality rates are high (95%–100%), some animals, particularly cattle and those with mild disease, can recover.*[19,27]

Pathologic Condition

- *The gross pathology of MCF varies considerably from severe multisystemic changes to complete absence of gross lesions, although oculonasal and oral lesions are most consistently present in all species.* A summary of the lesions of MCF in cattle and bison is presented as follows but readers should be directed to a complete review of the pathology of MCF for more information.[28] Gross lesions in terminally affected animals include oculonasal discharge, corneal edema, and erosive-ulcerative foci of the cornea, nasal planum, nasal sinus, oral cavity, oropharynx, trachea, esophagus, trachea, forestomachs, abomasum, cecum, colon, and urinary bladder.[28,29] Considerable hemorrhage is often concurrently present in the cecum, colon, and urinary bladder lesions. Some species differences in gross lesions occur; for example, generalized lymphadenomegaly is a consistent finding in cattle but is often underwhelming in bison, whereas myocardial necrosis is much more consistently observed in bison.[28] Exudative, wet, and crusting cutaneous lesions on the trunk, inguinal regions, perineum, and occasionally on the head and distal limbs can also be observed.
- *When present along with oculonasal and oral lesions, ulcerative and hemorrhagic cystitis in the urinary bladder is often sufficiently distinct enough to enable a tentative diagnosis of MCF.* Traumatic lesions from goring are quite common in terminally ill bison and should not be misconstrued as the cause of illness.[28]
- *The paramount histopathologic lesion is disseminated lymphocytic arteritis and phlebitis, affecting small-to-medium-sized vessels with variable necrosis of the vessel wall.* In chronic cases, vascular remodeling leads to proliferative changes most evident in medium-sized arteries.[19] Panophthalmitis, nonsuppurative encephalitis, lymphoid hyperplasia, and epithelial necrosis predominately in the gastrointestinal tract, multifocal bronchointerstitial pneumonia and lichenoid infiltration of the skin with folliculitis can also be observed in some cases.[28,29] Due to the variability of the presence of virus in affected tissues, testing of multiple different tissues is generally recommended.

- *Differential diagnoses include acute, severe bovine viral diarrhea virus and mucosal disease, foot and mouth disease, vesicular stomatitis, rinderpest, infectious bovine rhinotracheitis, enzootic hemorrhagic disease, and bluetongue.* Although the distribution of gross lesions in these other diseases typically differ from MCF, histopathology and ancillary diagnostic testing is often required to confidently exclude other causes (**Fig. 2**).

Diagnosis

Table 1 lists the most common assays for the detection of MCF viruses or antibodies with a brief indication of their utility and result interpretation. For some assays, submission of samples to a national reference or research laboratory is often necessary.

- *Definitive diagnosis of MCF requires the detection of MCF viruses in the blood or tissues of animals with compatible clinical signs and/or postmortem lesions.* Animals with clinical signs of MCF uniformly have detectable levels of virus in whole blood and tissue samples, which are easily detected by polymerase chain reaction (PCR). Although several PCR assays are available for MCF viruses predominately in research settings, standard or quantitative PCR for OvHV-2 are often the only diagnostic assay readily accessible to most North American practitioners. An OvHV-2-specific PCR[30,31] is sufficient to confirm most cases of MCF in cattle and bison in North America but can lead to misdiagnosis if the disease is caused by another MCF virus. It is critical that epidemiologic data, such as contact with reservoirs, be taken into consideration to choose the best PCR assay in different situations. For cases where the expected MCF virus is not detected, an MCF multiplex PCR or a herpesvirus consensus PCR should be used.[32,33] Recently, an OvHV-2 in situ hybridization (ISH) has been developed for the detection of viral components in association with lesions on tissues. Although this assay is useful to confirm SA-MCF in cattle and bison, it is especially valuable for confirming disease in sheep because asymptomatic or clinically infected animals and carrier animals cannot be distinguished by using standard PCR assays.[34] Virus isolation can be performed for certain MCF viruses, such as AlHV-1, but it is not possible for OvHV-2 due to the lack of an in vitro system to propagate the virus.
- *Detection of antibodies has no diagnostic value in clinical cases and is mostly used for the identification of infected carrier animals.* Cattle and bison can develop MCF before having time to mount a robust antibody response against the infecting MCF virus. A couple of serologic assays are available for the detection of MCF virus antibodies, including a competitive enzyme-linked immunosorbent assay (ELISA)[35] and immunoperoxidase test.

Control Management

- *Control and prevention of MCF centers on physical separation of MCF virus carriers from susceptible host species as there are no commercially available vaccines or effective therapies.* Long-range transmission at distance of greater than 3 miles has been documented and is not uncommonly observed in sporadic cases.[14] Although physical distance is paramount, other factors, such as predominant wind and environmental conditions should also be considered when evaluating transmission risk (see **Fig. 1**).

Although various treatments including corticosteroids have been attempted,[36,37] there is no evidence of their efficacy, and treatment of affected animals involves predominately supportive care.

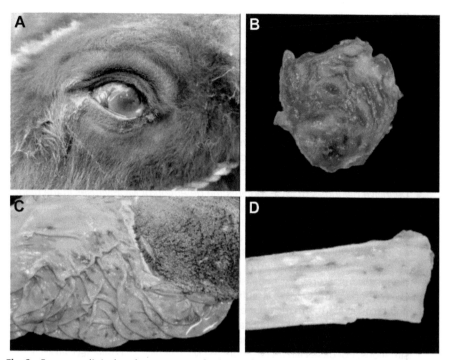

Fig. 2. Common clinical and postmortem findings of SA-MCF in cattle and bison. (*A*) Eye; peripheral corneal edema and conjunctivitis with catarrhal ocular discharge. Note that in MCF, corneal edema begins at the limbus and progresses centrally, in contrast to corneal edema observed in cases of bovine keratoconjunctivitis (*Moraxella* sp) and infectious bovine rhinotracheitis that typically begin from a central area of ulceration and progresses outward toward the limbus. (*B*) urinary bladder; multifocal ulcerative and hemorrhagic cystitis; (*C*) abomasum and rumen; multifocal ulcerative abomasitis and rumenitis; and (*D*) esophagus; multifocal ulcerative esophagitis.

Notification

MCF is listed as a monitored disease by the National List of Reportable Animal Diseases system, requiring that licensed veterinarians and veterinary laboratories report occurrence of disease to state and federal animal health officials.

BLUETONGUE VIRUS
Bluetongue Virus Etiology and Epidemiology

Bluetongue virus (BTV) is the causative agent of an arthropod-borne, noncontagious disease that primarily affects ruminant species. The virus is biologically transmitted by biting midges in the genus *Culicoides* that pick up the virus while taking a blood meal from an infected host and later spread the virus to naïve hosts when taking subsequent blood meals. Among domestic ruminant species, sheep present the most significant clinical disease, whereas infections of domestic cattle are typically subclinical. Among wild ruminants, white-tailed deer (*Odocoileus virginianus*) are most highly susceptible with significant morbidity and mortality. BTV has also been detected in pronghorn antelope (*Antilocapra americana*) and desert bighorn sheep (*Ovis canadensis*) in the United States. In Europe, during an outbreak of a particularly virulent BTV serotype (BTV-8), foreign to North America, captive European bison (*Bison bonasus*), North

Table 1
Common laboratory assays for malignant catarrhal fever

Goal	Sample Type	Assay	Interpretation
Detection of viral DNA	Fresh EDTA-blood; frozen buffy coat; and fresh or frozen tissues	MCFV-Specific Standard or quantitative PCR	Positive indicates infection with the MCFV tested. High levels in quantitative PCR are indicative of clinical disease.
	Fresh EDTA-blood; frozen buffy coat; and fresh or frozen tissues	Multiplex PCR (optimized to clinical animals)	Positive amplification is indicative of MCF with identification of the virus present. Specific for 6 MCFV.
	Fresh or frozen tissues (FFPE tissues may be used but the assay sensitivity will be reduced)	Herpesvirus Consensus PCR	Used when the MCF carriers are not identified or when a suspect case is negative by an MCFV specific PCR. Positive amplification is indicative of infection with a herpesvirus. Sequencing of the amplified DNA confirms virus identity.
	Formalin-fixed or FFPE tissues (<6 d in formalin)	OvHV-2 ISH	Positive reactivity associated with lesions confirms SA-MCF.
Detection of antibodies to MCFV	Fresh or frozen plasma or serum	ELISA and immune peroxidase test	Positive reaction indicates infection but does not distinguish the MCF virus. This is the test of choice to detect reservoirs but lacks any diagnostic value in clinical animals.
	Fresh or frozen serum	AlHV-1 virus neutralization	Detection of neutralizing antibodies. Specific to AlHV-1 only.

Abbreviations: AlHV-1, alcelaphine herpesvirus-1; EDTA-blood, blood collected with the anticoagulant ethylenediaminetetraacetic acid; ELISA, enzyme-linked immunosorbent assay; FFPE, formalin-fixed, paraffin-embedded; ISH, in situ hybridization; MCFV, malignant catarrhal fever viruses; PCR, polymerase chain reaction.

American bison (*Bison bison*), and yaks (*Bos grunniens grunniens*) showed clinical signs similar to sheep, with edema, conjunctivitis, and sudden death reported in all 3 species.

BTV is classified as an *Orbivirus* in the Reoviridae family and is characterized by a 10-segmented double-stranded RNA genome. The virus was first identified in the United States in 1948 in Texas and has since become endemic in the United States. Currently, there are 29 BTV serotypes recognized worldwide based on outer capsid serotype-specific neutralizing epitopes. Serotypes can differ with respect to virulence and the species of *Culicoides* midges able to transmit them. As of 2022, 17 serotypes are considered established or reported in the United States (BTV-1, 2, 3, 5, 6, 9, 10, 11, 12, 13, 14, 15, 17, 18, 19, 20, and 24).[38] The proliferation of serotypes is due to genetic drift and viral reassortment of the segmented genome in mammalian and insect hosts infected with multiple serotypes concurrently.[39]

Vector Biology and Ecology

Because of the noncontagious nature of BTV, virus transmission is limited by the presence of competent *Culicoides* species (Ceratopogonidae) and is therefore dependent on the biology and ecology of the insects and climate. Serotypes present in any given geographic area reflect the competent midge species populations in that area. The primary United States vector species of BTV in the central and western United States is *Culicoides sonorensis*. In the far southeastern United States, *Culicoides insignis* is also considered a competent BTV vector. It is likely that additional, unconfirmed vector species occur throughout the United States.[40] Female midges feed on the blood of vertebrate hosts to gather protein for egg development. Within the insect, the virus ingested in the blood meal from the infected animal must survive the hostile environment of the midge midgut, infect the epithelial cells of the midgut, escape the midgut, and infect the salivary glands where it can be passed to the next host during a subsequent blood feeding.

Culicoides are characterized by their extremely small size (1–3 mm total length) and by the unique wing patterns associated with each species, which are often used for morphologic identification. More than 1400 species of *Culicoides* midges have been named worldwide,[41] although relatively few of these are considered vectors of pathogens. In the United States, *C sonorensis* and *C insignis* are confirmed vectors of BTV, with several additional species suspected of transmitting the virus such as *Culicoides stellifer* and *Culicoides debilipalpis*.[40]

Culicoides progress through 4 life cycle stages: the egg, larva, pupa, and adult stages. Larval and pupal midges of most *Culicoides* species are considered semi-aquatic, often surviving along the banks of ponds, streams, springs, and other water bodies. Some midges occupy more specialized habitats, including tree-holes, manure piles, or rotting vegetation.[41] Highly organically enriched habitats are commonly used by many species, including the confirmed vector *C sonorensis*, the larvae of which are often found along the edges of dairy wastewater ponds. This vast range in habitats used by midge species underscores the difficulty in controlling these insects in their juvenile stages.

Most adult midges are crepuscular, with their peak activity occurring during dawn and dusk, although some midges are active throughout the night and during the day.[41] During periods of cold weather, midges may shift peak activity to warmer daylight hours. Although the active flight range of adult midges is generally considered relatively short (2–3 km maximum), there is evidence that midges may be picked up by air currents and passively transported hundreds of kilometers.[42]

Clinical Manifestation

Clinical BT disease is most significant in domestic sheep and white-tailed deer. In affected sheep, ulceration and hemorrhage of the mucous membranes of the upper gastrointestinal track (including the mouth) and nose are common. Swelling of the tongue and submandibular areas results in cyanosis of the tongue (hence, blue-tongue). Hyperemia of the coronary band is typically apparent and soreness in the hooves of the animal can lead to the characteristic arched stance of infected animals. Animals that survive infection may present as emaciated and lame and have increased susceptibility to secondary infection.

Pathologic Condition

Clinical signs of BT are attributed to damage of the vascular endothelium resulting from infection. Increased capillary permeability and intravascular coagulation results in edema, congestion, hemorrhage, inflammation, and necrosis of affected tissues. Animals become febrile and then develop edema of the lips, nose, face, and subman-dibular areas with excessive salivation and congestion in oral–nasal tissues, conjunc-tiva, and coronary bands, which leads to lameness. Animals will refuse to eat or drink due to the swelling and pain in their mouths. Peracute cases die within 7 to 9 days after exposure primarily due to severe pulmonary edema.

Diagnosis

Typical clinical signs can be used as a presumptive diagnosis, especially where the disease is endemic. Animals will develop a serologic response in 7 to 14 days after exposure, which can be detected by agar gel immunodiffusion (known to cross-react with antibodies to other orbiviruses, such as epizootic hemorrhagic disease vi-rus) and competitive ELISA. Identification of BTV in blood samples is based on virus isolation using cell culture or in embryonated chicken eggs and by PCR. Whole genome sequencing methods are recommended for virus characterization to better understand virus dynamics, evolution, and spread, including reassortment events that may lead to changes in virulence. Postmortem examination will show hemor-rhages and necrosis of capillaries in the cheek and esophageal mucosa, subcutane-ous and intermuscular edema and hemorrhaging, myocardial and intestinal hemorrhages, necrosis particularly in the papillary muscle of the left ventricle, and pneumonia.

Control and Management

There is no specific treatment of BTV-infected animals aside from supportive care, such as soft food, good husbandry, and forced hydration when necessary. Attenuated BTV vaccines are in use in some parts of the world, although these attenuated vac-cines carry risks of reversion to virulence, reassortment with wild-type virus, and the ability to cross placental barriers and cause fetal death or injury. The only North Amer-ican attenuated BTV vaccine currently approved is for BTV-10 in sheep in California. Important to recognize, South African vaccines can target up to 5 serotypes in a single dose.[39] Various recombinant, subunit, and nanoparticle vaccines that avoid the pitfalls of attenuated vaccines are being developed but are not yet commercially available. Killed BTV vaccines are often used in response to outbreaks but require multiple doses for protective immunity, and it is short-lived.

In the absence of approved vaccines, vector and animal management practices can be used to prevent infection. If possible, moving sick animals indoors can prevent biting midges from spreading the virus to additional hosts. In situations where moving animals indoors is impractical or undesirable, vector habitat management methods can be used. Efforts should be made to minimize overfilling of water troughs or leaking irrigation pipes that lead to moist soil in the surrounding area, and proper manure management, especially around established water bodies, is critical. Chemical control can also be used to manage adult biting midge populations, including environmental spraying, insecticide-impregnated mesh or screening, and insecticide pour-ons or dunks, although the efficacy of many chemical agents against adult midges has not been fully investigated.[43]

Notification

BTV is considered a reportable disease in the United States by the USDA APHIS. Currently, BTV-8 is considered a notifiable disease in the United States, whereas the remaining serotypes are monitored by the USDA APHIS.[44] BTV is also listed as a reportable disease by the World Organisation for Animal Health (WOAH), which monitors diseases globally.

NEW WORLD SCREWWORM: A CONTINUING THREAT TO US AGRICULTURE, WILDLIFE, AND PUBLIC HEALTH
Introduction/History/Definitions/Background

New World Screwworm (NWS), *Cochliomyia hominivorax* (Coquerel), is an obligate parasite of warm-blooded animals and originally endemic in warm areas of the western hemisphere (**Fig. 3**).

This parasite was first identified in 1858 by the French naval physician, Dr Charles Coquerel, who described it from observation in the nasal passages and buccal cavities of several prisoners incarcerated at the penal colony of Cayenne in French Guiana.[45] Coquerel was sent to determine the cause of death of prisoners being eaten alive by maggots. Coquerel discovered it was a species of fly, new to science, and named it *Lucilia hominivorax*. *Lucilia* meaning "shiny" and *hominivorax* meaning "man-eater."

Until the research of Emory C. Cushing and Walter S. Patton, the taxonomy of the screwworm was misunderstood. They discovered that the screwworm that livestock producers and others had been trying to control was 2 species that closely resembled each other. One, *C hominivorax*, a primary obligate parasite, was pathogenic and fed on the living tissue of the host. The other species, *Cochliomyia macellaria* Fabricius,[46] was the more common and benign facultative parasite, and fed on necrotic tissue.

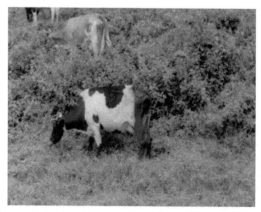

Fig. 3. New World Screwworm larvae have penetrated the vascular system of a cow, resulting in uncontrolled hemorrhaging.

Although the taxonomic nomenclature continued to be in a state of change, this discovery helped lead to the most successful eradication program in the history of medical and veterinary entomology.[47]

Any wound or bodily orifice is a susceptible site for the gravid female fly to lay an egg mass of about 200 to 300 eggs, which are glued to the animal in a shingle-like pattern.[46] The eggs generally hatch in 10 to 12 hours and the almost microscopic (about 0.03 inches or 0.762 millimeters) first instar larvae (maggots) enter the wound or burrow into soft mucosal tissue, initiating the myiasis or infestation. Once a wound is infested, it gives off an odor attractive to other NWS flies looking for a site to lay their eggs, which can result in reinfestations with thousands of larvae feeding in the wound. The larvae feed for approximately 5 to 7 days on the tissue, blood, and sera produced by using their 2 sharp, heavily sclerotized mouth hooks to scrape into the living tissue of the host. The larvae pass through 2 molts, growing to more than 0.5 inches or 1.27 centimeters in length, and then exit the wound, drop to the ground and burrow into the soil where they form the pupal stage. Flies emerge in about 7 days and crawl to the surface and onto the surrounding vegetation. Flies are ready to mate in approximately 2 to 3 days. Female NWS flies generally only mate once and males may mate around 10 times. Females may live up to 30 days and may lay an egg mass once every 3 days.[48] The life cycle is completed in approximately 3 weeks.[47] NWS flies occur in relatively low numbers when compared with C macellaria and other insects.[49]

Incorporating the previous results of both field observations and research on NWS, Edward F. Knipling and Raymond C. Bushland, working together with their teams, developed and refined what was known as the sterile male technique, now known as the sterile insect technique (SIT), and its use to eradicate NWS. Knipling thought of the concept,[50,51] and Bushland was primarily involved with developing the original protocols to mass rear[52,53] NWS flies and to sterilize the insects while preserving their quality and competitiveness with wild sterile flies.[54] Currently, there are at least 32 countries with SIT programs, and there are 29 species of insects being targeted by the technique.[55–57]

Using the SIT, NWS has been eradicated from approximately 1.7 million square miles or 4.4 million square kilometers, initially in the United States and then with cooperative binational agreements with other countries, by the USDA–Screwworm Eradication program. New World Screwworm was eradicated from the southeastern United States (1959), southwestern United States (1966), Mexico (1991), Belize and Guatemala (1994), El Salvador, (1995), Honduras (1996), Nicaragua (1999), Costa Rica (2000), and Panama (2008).[57]

Discussion

Concern
After the success of the NWS eradication programs, what is the concern? The concern is the very real probability of reintroduction of NWS into the United States or other NWS-free areas. Reintroductions into NWS-free areas have occurred several times, resulting in outbreaks, each with associated losses and expenses. Outbreaks have occurred in the United States, Texas (1968, 1972, 1975); Libya (1990); Mexico (1992, 1993); Mexico (2001–2002, 2003) Panama (2003), Aruba (2004, 2011); Panama (2009, 2012); United States, Florida (2016–2017); Panama (2022–2023); and Costa Rica (2023). Vigilance and the timely submission of myiasis samples to the State Animal Health Official (SAHO) or USDA APHIS official will help protect the United States from future outbreaks.

Transport of New World screwworm-infested animals

Transport of infested animals is the most common movement of screwworm from an infested geographic area to a screwworm-free area. This may occur in a relatively local area, such as movement of infested livestock in a truck from one farm to another, or movement of an infested pet from one country to another, such as movement of an infested dog from Venezuela to the United States via commercial airline. The source of a screwworm outbreak in Libya was traced back to Uruguay. This long-distance transport was via a ship transporting thousands of sheep, some with NWS myiasis. If screwworm populations are present, screwworms can potentially be transported to anywhere on the planet in a relatively short period. In relation to the United States, there have been 29 known detections/introductions from 1986 to 2019. States involved are as follows: Florida (21 incidents); Texas (2); New York (2); and Colorado, Connecticut, Mississippi, Alabama, Utah, and the Territory of Puerto Rico, each with one incident. The numbers do not add up to 29 because some cases passed through Florida undetected. Countries of origin of infested animals include Argentina (15 incidents); Venezuela (4); Panama (3); and Honduras, Brazil, Cuba, Trinidad, Colombia, Dominican Republic, and unknown (Florida 2016–2017 outbreak), each with one incident. Species involved were horses (16); dogs (7); humans (3); cat (1); and unknown (Florida 2016–2017 outbreak). To date, the main pathways of introduction have been horses from Argentina (15 times) and dogs (2 times) from Venezuela, resulting in an update to United States import regulations to require horses, ruminants, and swine, as well as dogs, imported from regions of the world where screwworm is considered to exist to be inspected and treated prior to export as well as on import, if necessary, for screwworm, with related health certificate declarations to prevent the introduction of screwworm to the United States. (USDA APHIS 9 CFR Part 93 Subparts C, D, E, and F).

Screwworm myiasis in wildlife

Screwworm myiasis in wildlife is not easily observed but, when present, occurs continuously and at different levels, depending in part on host life cycles during the year.[58] Those species in which screwworm myiasis has been verified in the United States include Texas cottontail rabbits, *Sylvilagus floridanus champmani* Allen; Texas jack rabbit, *Lepus californicus texianus* Waterhouse; Texas opossum, *Didelphis mesamericana texensis* Allen; and white-tailed deer, *O virginianus texanus* Mearns[58] (**Fig. 4**).

Impact of screwworm on wild hosts in the tropics is even less visible due to the complexity of the environment and general avoidance of humans by wild animals. In 1987, during the 11-year period that JB Welch worked on screwworm in the Republic of Panama, a freshly collected carcass of a howler monkey, *Alouatta* sp, from the area of the Panama Canal, had a wound on one of its biceps that was infested with screwworm, *C hominivorax*.[54]

In early July 2016, several Florida Key deer, *O virginianus clavicum* (an endangered subspecies of the white-tailed deer), within the National Key Deer Refuge in Big Pine and Little Pine Keys, Florida, presented with screwworm myiasis and were euthanized. As it was rutting season, males were fighting for the right to mate and the number of wounds (egg-laying sites) and infestations rapidly increased (**Fig. 5**).

The USDA, the Florida Department of Agriculture and Consumer Services, and the US Fish and Wildlife Services worked cooperatively along with other agencies and individuals to eradicate the outbreak using sterile flies that came from the sterile fly mass production facility from the Panama–United States Commission for the Eradication and Prevention of Screwworm in Pacora, Republic of Panama. A total of 135 deer were euthanized before the end of the outbreak, and it was estimated that for every

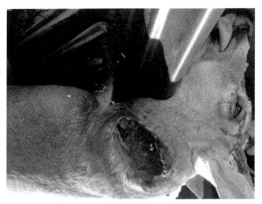

Fig. 4. A Florida Key deer buck with a neck wound infested with hundreds of third instar New World Screwworm (NWS) larvae and approximately 9 NWS egg masses. This photo illustrates the extreme damage NWS myiasis can cause.

deer euthanized, another died in the field. In addition to the deer, one raccoon, *Procyon lotor* (Linnaeus), was collected with screwworm myiasis during the outbreak.[59] A recent publication reported that 27 of 618 feral hogs, *Sus scrofa* Linnaeus, harvested in the Department of Artigas, Uruguay, during a 3-year period (2017–2020) were positive for screwworm myiasis.[60] The publication stated that the location of the wounds appeared to suggest they were caused by aggressive behavior between adult males.[60] There was no report of NWS myiasis in *Bison bison* Linnaeas, the American bison or buffalo.

Point of care

Treatment of wounds and collection of larval samples should follow the veterinary protocol for the treatment of myiasis, with a couple of changes if the myiasis is suspicious or NWS is suspected. Ten or more larvae should be collected from various locations and depths within the wound. Larvae should be placed in a collection tube or jar and filled with either 70% or (preferably) 95% ethanol (for DNA and molecular analysis). After the sample has been collected for submission and identification, the wound should

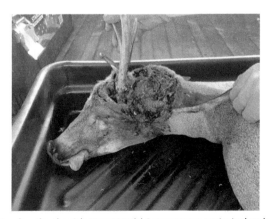

Fig. 5. A Florida Key deer buck with New World Screwworm myiasis that has destroyed most of the soft tissue of the Key deer's head.

be treated with an approved insecticide and all larvae removed from the wound. It must be assured that all larvae are killed and not just placed in the trash. If euthanasia of the host is required, ensure that all larvae are killed.[61]

Critical importance to report

NWS has been designated by the USDA (https://www.aphis.usda.gov/aphis/ourfocus/animalhealth/monitoring-and-surveillance/nlrad/ct_national_list_reportable_animal_diseases) and the World Organisation for Animal Health (WOAH) (formerly OIE) as a reportable disease. Reporting NWS myiasis is mandatory. The State and Federal Animal Health Officials should be contacted immediately and the sample should be shipped as quickly as possible to the National Veterinary Services Laboratory in Ames, Iowa for official identification.[61,62] If a wound is thought to be infested with NWS larvae, additional information may be found at http://www.aphis.usda.gov/index.shtml, and then by typing "screwworm" in the search box.

Summary (New World screwworm)

The NWS continues to injure and kill animals in endemic areas. Livestock, companion animals, wildlife, and humans serve as potential hosts, and any wound or bodily orifice can serve as a site for females to lay their egg masses, which could then lead to myiasis. Untreated myiasis can lead to the death of the host. NWS myiasis is a reportable disease and must be reported to your State and Federal Animal Health Officials. Please do not transport animals with myiasis; although NWS has been eradicated, vigilance must be continued to help protect the United States from NWS reintroduction and outbreaks. In addition to the vigilance of State and Federal veterinarians and wildlife managers, private veterinarians and their clients must also understand that NWS is a real and continuing threat to US agriculture, wildlife, and public health.

SUMMARY

Maintaining an awareness of the risks and clinical presentations of the 3 reemerging and notifiable diseases to watch, MCF, BTV, and NWS, is essential to protecting cattle and bison in North America, as well as other susceptible animals, including, in the case of NWS, humans. Global changes in climate will alter the established epidemiology of many diseases of consequence, including those discussed in this article such as BTV, biological vectors, and hosts. Changes may be noted with vector competence, local and long-distance dispersal dynamics and increased transmission period duration with earlier spring onset and later fall transmission, among others (Hudson 2023). Importantly, when clinical signs are suggestive of MCF, BTV, or NWS, immediately contact your State and Federal Animal Health Officials to report your findings to initiate confirmation and an appropriate response to help protect North American cattle and bison, other susceptible animals, and humans by preventing establishment and spread of diseases that pose potential risks and losses to production, the health and sometimes life of the animal, and to the livelihoods of producers.

CLINICS CARE POINTS

- Control and prevention of MCF centers on physical separation of MCF virus carriers from susceptible host species as there are no commercially available vaccines or effective therapies.

- The presence of ulcerative and hemorrhagic cystitis in the urinary bladder along with oculonasal and oral lesions, is often sufficiently distinct enough to enable a tentative diagnosis of MCF.
- Detection of antibodies has no diagnostic value in clinical cases and is mostly used for the identification of infected carrier animals.
- There is no specific treatment of BTV-infected animals aside from supportive care, such as soft food, good husbandry, and forced hydration when necessary.
- BTV transmission is limited by the presence of competent Culicoides species and is therefore dependent on the biology and ecology of the insects and climate.
- BTV-infected sheep present the most significant clinical disease, whereas infections of domestic cattle are typically subclinical. Among wild ruminants, white-tailed deer (Odocoileus virginianus) are most highly susceptible with significant morbidity and mortality.
- Only one BT vaccine is available in the United States and only protects against serotype 10, is only approved for use in California, and only for sheep. In the absence of approved vaccines, vector and animal management practices can be used to prevent infection, including appropriate use of insecticides and minimizing wet and humid habitats, such as with water-soaked soils near water troughs or leaking irrigation pipes, where Culicoides larvae and pupae tend to develop.
- Be alert that NWS gravid female flies lay their egg mass of 200 to 300 eggs glued to the animal in a shingle-like pattern in any wound or bodily orifice, hatching as larvae feeding on live tissue of the wound.
- Although NWS was eradicated from the United States by 1966, there is a constant real probability of reintroduction of NWS into the United States or other NWS-free areas. Reintroductions into NWS-free areas continue to occur, each with associated losses and expenses, including the United States with 29 known detections/ introductions from 1986 to 2019. Heightened vigilance is essential.
- NWS-infected species associated with reintroductions have involved horses, dogs, humans, a cat, and an unknown (Florida 2016-2017 outbreak).
- Transport of NWS-infested animals is the primary mode of movement of NWS from an infested geographic area to a screwworm-free area.
- Treatment of wounds and collection of larval samples should follow the veterinary protocol for the treatment of myiasis, with a couple of changes if the myiasis is suspicious or NWS is suspected. Ten or more larvae should be collected from various locations and depths within the wound. Larvae should be placed in a collection tube or jar and filled with either 70% or (preferably) 95% ethanol (for DNA and molecular analysis) for laboratory examination.
- After the myiasis sample has been collected for submission and identification, the wound should be treated with an approved insecticide and all larvae removed from the wound. It must be assured that all larvae are killed and not just placed in the trash. If euthanasia of the host is required, ensure that all larvae present on the animal are removed and killed.

DISCLOSURE

The authors have nothing to disclose and have no known conflicts of interest.

REFERENCES

1. Davison AJ, Eberle R, Ehlers B, et al. The order Herpesvirales. Arch Virol 2009; 154(1):171-7.
2. Li H, Gailbreath K, Flach EJ, et al. A novel subgroup of rhadinoviruses in ruminants. J Gen Virol 2005;86(11):3021-6.

3. Li H, Cunha CW, Taus NS, et al. Malignant catarrhal fever: inching toward understanding. Annu Rev Anim Biosci 2014;2:209–33.

4. Li H, Snowder G, O'Toole D, et al. Transmission of ovine herpesvirus 2 in lambs. J Clin Microbiol 1998;36(1):223–6.

5. Li H, Shen DT, Jessup DA, et al. Prevalence of antibody to malignant catarrhal fever virus in wild and domestic ruminants by competitive-inhibition ELISA. J Wildl Dis 1996;32(3):437–43.

6. Li H, Shen DT, O'Toole D, et al. Investigation of sheep-associated malignant catarrhal fever virus infection in ruminants by PCR and competitive inhibition enzyme-linked immunosorbent assay. J Clin Microbiol 1995;33(8):2048–53.

7. Li H, Snowder G, O'Toole D, et al. Transmission of ovine herpesvirus 2 among adult sheep. Vet Microbiol 2000;71(1–2):27–35.

8. Li H, Snowder G, Crawford TB. Production of malignant catarrhal fever virus-free sheep. Vet Microbiol 1999;65(2):167–72.

9. Stirewalt DL, Pogosova-Agadjanyan EL, Khalid N, et al. Single-stranded linear amplification protocol results in reproducible and reliable microarray data from nanogram amounts of starting RNA. Genomics 2004;83(2):321–31.

10. Li H, Taus NS, Lewis GS, et al. Shedding of ovine herpesvirus 2 in sheep nasal secretions: the predominant mode for transmission. J Clin Microbiol 2004; 42(12):5558–64.

11. Berezowski JA, Appleyard GD, Crawford TB, et al. An outbreak of sheep-associated malignant catarrhal fever in bison (Bison bison) after exposure to sheep at a public auction sale. J Vet Diagn Invest 2005;17(1):55–8.

12. Li H, Taus NS, Jones C, et al. A devastating outbreak of malignant catarrhal fever in a bison feedlot. J Vet Diagn Invest 2006;18(1):119–23.

13. Müller-Doblies UU, Egli J, Li H, et al. [Malignant catarrhal fever in Switzerland. 1.Epidemiology]. Schweiz Arch Tierheilkd 2001;143(4):173–83.

14. Li H, Karney G, O'Toole D, et al. Long distance spread of malignant catarrhal fever virus from feedlot lambs to ranch bison. Can Vet J 2008;49(2):183–5.

15. Mushi EZ, Rurangirwa FR. Epidemiology of bovine malignant catarrhal fevers, a review. Vet Res Commun 1981;5(2):127–42.

16. Rossiter PB, Jessett DM, Karstad L. Role of wildebeest fetal membranes and fluids in the transmission of malignant catarrhal fever virus. Vet Rec 1983; 113(7):150–2.

17. Taus NS, Oaks JL, Gailbreath K, et al. Experimental aerosol infection of cattle (Bos taurus) with ovine herpesvirus 2 using nasal secretions from infected sheep. Vet Microbiol 2006;116(1–3):29–36.

18. Gailbreath KL, O'Toole D, Taus NS, et al. Experimental nebulization of American bison (Bison bison) with low doses of ovine herpesvirus 2 from sheep nasal secretions. Vet Microbiol 2010;143(2–4):389–93.

19. O'Toole D, Li H, Miller D, et al. Chronic and recovered cases of sheep-associated malignant catarrhal fever in cattle. Vet Rec 1997;140(20):519–24.

20. Schultheiss PC, Collins JK, Austgen LE, et al. Malignant catarrhal fever in bison, acute and chronic cases. J Vet Diagn Invest 1998;10(3):255–62.

21. O'Toole D, Li H, Sourk C, et al. Malignant catarrhal fever in a bison (Bison bison) feedlot, 1993-2000. J Vet Diagn Invest 2002;14(3):183–93.

22. Plowright W. Malignant catarrhal fever virus. In: Dinter Z, Morein B, editors. Virus infections of ruminants. 1st edition. New York: Elsevier Science Publishers BV; 1990. p. 123–50.

23. Smith BP. Malignant Catarrhal Fever (bovine malignant catarrh; malignant head catarrh). In: Smith BP, editor. Large animal internal medicine. 2nd edition. St. Louis: Mosby; 1996. p. 814–7.
24. Brown CC, Baker DC, Barker IK. Alimentary system. In: Maxie MG, editor. Jubb, Kennedy and Palmer's pathology of domestic animals. 5th edition., vol. 2. Edinburgh: Saunders Elsevier; 2007. p. 1–296.
25. Russell GC, Stewart JP, Haig DM. Malignant catarrhal fever: a review. Vet J 2009; 179(3):324–35.
26. Mitchell ESE, Scholes SFE. Unusual presentation of malignant catarrhal fever involving neurological disease in young calves. Vet Rec 2009;164(8):240–2.
27. Hamilton AF. Account of three outbreaks of malignant catarrhal fever in cattle in the Republic of Ireland. Vet Rec 1990;127(9):231–2.
28. O'Toole D, Li H. The pathology of malignant catarrhal fever, with an emphasis on ovine herpesvirus 2. Vet Pathol 2014;51(2):437–52.
29. Maxie MG, editor. Jubb, Kennedy and Palmer's pathology of domestic animals. 5th edition, vol. 2. Edinburgh: Saunders Elsevier; 2007.
30. Baxter SI, Pow I, Bridgen A, et al. PCR detection of the sheep-associated agent of malignant catarrhal fever. Arch Virol 1993;132(1–2):145–59.
31. Traul DL, Taus NS, Oaks JL, et al. Validation of non-nested and real-time PCR for diagnosis of sheep-associated malignant catarrahal fever in clinical samples. J Vet Diagn Invest 2007;19(4):405–8.
32. Cunha CW, Otto L, Taus NS, et al. Development of a multiplex real-time PCR for detection and differentiation of malignant catarrhal fever viruses in clinical samples. J Clin Microbiol 2009;47(8):2586–9.
33. VanDevanter DR, Warrener P, Bennett L, et al. Detection and analysis of diverse herpesviral species by consensus primer PCR. J Clin Microbiol 1996;34(7): 1666–71.
34. Pesavento PA, Cunha CW, Li H, et al. In Situ hybridization for localization of ovine herpesvirus 2, the agent of sheep-associated malignant catarrhal fever, in formalin-fixed tissues. Vet Pathol 2019;56(1):78–86.
35. Li H, McGuire TC, Müller-Doblies UU, et al. A simpler, more sensitive competitive inhibition ELISA for detection of antibody to malignant catarrhal fever viruses. J Vet Diagn Invest 2001;13(4):361–4.
36. Milne EM, Reid HW. Recovery of a cow from malignant catarrhal fever. Vet Rec 1990;126(26):640–1.
37. Penny C. Recovery of cattle from malignant catarrhal fever. Vet Rec 1998; 142(9):227.
38. Bluetongue. United States Department of Agriculture Animal and Plant Health Inspection Service (USDA APHIS). 2022. Available at: http://www.aphis.usda.gov/aphis/ourfocus/animalhealth/animal-disease-information/cattle-disease-information/bluetongue-disease-info/index.
39. Drolet BS, McGregor BL, Cohnstaedt LW, et al. Reoviridae. In: McVey DS, Kennedy M, Chengappa MM, et al, editors. Veterinary microbiology. 4th edition. Hoboken, NJ: John Wiley & Sons Inc; 2022. p. 679–92.
40. McGregor BL, Shults PT, McDermott EG. A review of the vector status of North American Culicoides (Diptera: Ceratopogonidae) for Bluetongue Virus, Epizootic Hemorrhagic Disease Virus, and other arboviruses of concern. Curr Trop Med Rep 2022;9(4):130–9.
41. Mellor PS, Boorman J, Baylis M. Culicoides biting midges: their role as arbovirus vectors. Annu Rev Entomol 2000;45:307–40.

42. Jacquet S, Huber K, Pagès N, et al. Range expansion of the Bluetongue vector, Culicoides imicola, in continental France likely due to rare wind-transport events. Sci Rep 2016;6:27247.

43. Carpenter S, Mellor PS, Torr SJ. Control techniques for Culicoides biting midges and their application in the U.K. and northwestern Palaearctic. Med Vet Entomol 2008;22(3):175–87.

44. National List of Reportable Animal Diseases. United States Department of Agriculture Animal and Plant Health Inspection Service (USDA APHIS). 2023. Available at: https://www.aphis.usda.gov/aphis/ourfocus/animalhealth/monitoring-and-surveillance/nlrad/ct_national_list_reportable_animal_diseases.

45. Coquerel C. Note sur des larves apartenant a une espece niouvelle de diptere (Lucilia hominivorax) developees dans les sinus frontaux de l'homme a Cayenne. Annales Societe Entomologique de France 1858;27:171–6.

46. Cushing EC, Patton WS. Studies on the higher Diptera of medical and veterinary importance, Cochliomyia americana sp. nov., the screw-worm fly of the New World. Ann Trop J Med Parasitol 1933;27:539–51.

47. Laake EW, Cushing EC, Parish HE. Biology of the primary screw worm fly, Cochliomyia americana, and a comparison of its stages with those of C. macellaria. United States Department of Agriculture; 1936. p. 1–24. USDA Technical Bulletin No. 500.

48. Thomas DB, Mangan RL. Oviposition and wound-visiting behavior of the screw-worm fly, Cochliomyia hominivorax (Diptera: Calliphoridae). Ann Entomol Soc Am 1989;82(4):526–34.

49. Lindquist AW. A study of the incidence and habits of Cochliomyia americana by means of flytraps. J Kans Entomol Soc 1938;11(3):97–204.

50. Knipling EF. Possibilities of insect control or eradication through the use of sexually sterile males. J Econ Entomol 1955;48(4):459–62.

51. Knipling EF. Control of screw-worm fly by atomic radiation. Sci Mon 1957;85(4):195–202.

52. Melvin R, Bushland RC. A method of rearing Cochliomyia americana C. & P. on artificial media88. U.S. Bureau of Entomology and Plant Quarantine; 1936. p. 1–2.

53. Melvin R, Bushland RC. The nutritional requirements for screwworm larvae. J Econ Entomol 1940;33(6):850–2.

54. Bushland RC, Hopkins DE. Sterilization of screw-worm flies with x-rays and gamma rays. J Econ Entomol 1953;46(4):648–56.

55. Klassen W, Curtis CF, Hendrichs J. Chapter 1. History of the Sterile Insect Technique. Abstract. In Sterile Insect Technique, 2nd Edition. CRC Press. 2021. p. 2.

56. International Atomic Energy Agency. Nuclear Applications for Insect Pest Control. History of Transboundary Shipments of Sterile Insects. Table of Transboundary Shipments of Sterile Insects. p. 1.

57. Wyss JH. Screwworm eradication in the Americas. Ann N Y Acad Sci 2000;916:186–93. Hoboken, NJ: John Wiley & Sons Inc.

58. Lindquist AW. Myiasis in wild animals in southwestern Texas. J Econ Entomol 1937;30(5):735–40.

59. United States Department of Agriculture Veterinary Services (USDA VS). Final report for the APHIS Veterinary Services response to the 2016–2017 outbreak of New World Screwworm (NWS) in Florida. Available at: https://www.aphis.usda.gov/animal_health/emergency_management/downloads/public-nws-usdaaphis-final-report.pdf. 2017;1-34.

60. Altuna M, Hickner PV, Castro G, et al. New World Screwworm (Cochliomyia hominivorax) myiasis in feral swine of Uruguay: One Health and transboundary disease implications. Parasites Vectors 2021;14(1):26.
61. United States Department of Agriculture Animal and Plant Health Inspection Service (USDA APHIS). The Foreign Animal Disease preparedness and response plan (FAD PReP)—disease response strategy: New World Screwworm Myiasis. Available at: https://www.aphis.usda.gov/animal_health/emergency_management/downloads/nws_myiasis_disease_strategy.pdf. 2018;1-25.
62. United States Department of Agriculture Animal and Plant Health Inspection Service (USDA APHIS). Foreign Animal Disease preparedness and response plan (FAD PReP)—APHIS Foreign Animal Disease framework: Roles and communication. Available at: https://www.aphis.usda.gov/animal_health/emergency_management/downloads/documents_manuals/fadprep_manual_1.pdf. 2022;1-87.

Rinderpest
A Disease of the Past, and a Present Threat

Mariana Marrana, DVM[a],
Muhammad Javed Arshed, DVM, MSc, PhD[b,1],
Mo Salman, DVM, MPVM, PhD[b,c],*

KEYWORDS

- Rinderpest • Transboundary animal diseases • Bovine diseases
- Eradicated pathogen • Biothreat

KEY POINTS

- Rinderpest is a highly contagious viral disease that affects ungulates such as cattle, buffalo, yak, and various wildlife species, leading to significant morbidity and mortality.
- The global eradication of rinderpest was successfully accomplished in 2011 through extensive vaccination efforts.
- Today, safeguarding against the re-emergence of rinderpest in animal populations is paramount.
- The Food and Agriculture Organization of the United Nations and the World Organisation for Animal Health (formerly OIE) are entrusted through a series of resolutions with the responsibility to prevent the re-emergence of rinderpest in animals.
- The primary defense against its resurgence lies in maintaining the awareness of this disease and implementation of the *Global rinderpest action plan—posteradication* to rapidly respond to a potential re-emergence through rapidly deployable diagnostic tests and vaccines.

BACKGROUND AND HISTORY

For centuries, outbreaks of rinderpest (RP) wrought havoc, causing the demise of millions of cattle, buffalo, yak, and wildlife across 3 continents. RP killed 80% to 90% of Africa's cattle in the late 1800s and early 1900s, which translated to hundreds of millions of head, and caused heavy losses in Asia, the Middle East, and Europe.[1] This

[a] Preparedness and Resilience Department, World Organisation for Animal Health, 12 Rue de Prony, Paris 75017, France; [b] Food and Agriculture Organization of the UN Viale delle Terme di Caracalla, 00153 Rome, Italy; [c] Animal Population Health Institute of College of Veterinary Medicine and Biomedical Sciences, Colorado State University, Mail stop 1644, APHI, CVMBS, CSU, Fort Collins, CO 80523-1644, USA
[1] Present address: House 5, Street, 6, Royal Avenue, Lane 10, Park Road, Islamabad, Pakistan.
* Corresponding author. Food and Agriculture Organization of the United Nations, Rome, Italy.
E-mail address: mo.salman@colostate.edu

Vet Clin Food Anim 40 (2024) 337–343
https://doi.org/10.1016/j.cvfa.2024.01.008
0749-0720/24/© 2024 Elsevier Inc. All rights reserved.

devastation led to widespread famine, starvation, and the crippling inability of hundreds of communities to utilize draft animals for agricultural tasks, irrigation, and transportation. A large outbreak of RP triggered the Great Ethiopian Famine of 1888 to 1892, where millions of people died of starvation.[1] This disease led to the establishment of the World Organisation for Animal Health (WOAH; formerly OIE) following the introduction of the virus to Europe in 1920 through the importation of cattle from India. It should be noticed that this disease has never been reported in the United States.

RP is a highly contagious disease that afflicts even toed ungulates such as cattle, buffalo, yak, and various wildlife species, causing significant morbidity and mortality. The disease typically manifests as the "stomatitis-enteritis syndrome," marked by erosive oral lesions and diarrhea. However, the severity of clinical signs varies based on the specific RP virus strain, as well as the host species and breed.[2]

Global eradication of RP was achieved through widespread vaccination of cattle using live attenuated RP vaccines, notably the thermostable vaccine developed by Dr. Walter Plowright in 1957. This effort was coupled with rigorous sero-monitoring of vaccinated animals and extensive surveillance to confirm the absence of RP after vaccination efforts ceased.[1] RP remains a listed disease by the WOAH, which requires immediate notification should it be detected by a member country.[3]

From the late 1990s up to the early 2000s, there were numerous national, regional, and continental control and eradication programs for RP. These programs had the added benefit of fostering the development of veterinary services, laboratories, and veterinary schools in regions that were previously underserved, in an effort to increase production of livestock and food and stimulate national economies.[1,4] The first coordinated international control program for RP was implemented from 1963 to 1975 in Africa. The Inter-African Bureau of Epizootic Diseases was founded in 1950 with a plan to eliminate RP from Africa. Other programs such as the multi-nation joint project (JP15), the Pan African Programme of the Control of Epizootics, and the Pan African Rinderpest Campaign were implemented in Africa, while separate initiatives successfully eradicated RP from the Asian continent. The final push for eradication was the Global Rinderpest Eradication Program, led by the Food and Agriculture Organization of the United Nations (FAO), which started in 1994 and set 2010 as the deadline for eradication. The FAO tirelessly collaborated with numerous national, regional, and international partners, including WOAH, which was in charge of assessing countries' dossiers for official recognition of freedom from the disease. Their collective efforts culminated in the monumental achievement of eradicating RP from animal populations worldwide. The last case of RP was reported in 2001, in Kenya, and RP was jointly declared as eradicated by FAO and WOAH in May 2011.[1,5]

Today, safeguarding against the re-emergence of RP in animal populations is paramount. It is a matter of utmost importance for animal health, global economies, and worldwide food security. The FAO and the WOAH are actively involved in coordinating the process of sequestration and destruction of RP virus (RPV) containing material (RVCM). Several institutes worldwide still retain RVCM, as defined in the WOAH Terrestrial Animal Health Code, including vaccines. These, in addition to synthetic reconstruction of the virus, are the only possible sources of virus reintroduction into susceptible animals.[6] Therefore, the member countries should not manipulate existing RVCM, or synthesize or produce RVCM, unless authorized by FAO and WOAH. The FAO and the WOAH are entrusted through a series of resolutions with the responsibility to prevent the re-emergence of RP in animals. Their duties encompass promoting adherence to such resolutions that include the destruction and sequestration of RVCM in laboratories designated by the FAO and the WOAH for their purpose. Some of these facilities hold the global reserve of RP vaccine, which would be accessible in an emergency cause by RP re-emergence. Some FAO–WOAH-designated RP holding facilities are also FAO/WOAH reference laboratories for RP. Should a case of RP be suspected, these are the only laboratories in the world that can perform case confirmation.[3]

It has been more than 20 years since RP was last observed by farmers or veterinarians in the field. The primary defense against its resurgence lies in maintaining the awareness of this disease and having a tried and tested plan to rapidly respond to a potential re-emergence. To achieve this goal, the Global Rinderpest Action Plan (GRAP) was devised, tested, and regularly updated through collaborative efforts by the FAO and the WOAH. The FAO–WOAH Joint Rinderpest Secretariat spearheaded the development of the GRAP.[7] This document complements national, regional, and continental contingency plans for RP. It outlines the roles and responsibilities of all relevant stakeholders in the 5 stages of the emergency management cycle. It also includes the deployment framework for the global RP vaccine reserve.

DISEASE CHARACTERISTICS
Etiology

RP is caused by a negative-strand RNA virus of the Morbillivirus genus within the family Paramyxoviridae.[2] The virus existed as a single serotype, so that all strains cross-protect fully and are only differentiated by molecular characterization. It is closely related to viruses causing *peste des petits ruminants* (PPR), canine distemper, and measles. RPV is heat sensitive and can survive for 48 hours in infected premises.

Transmission

RPV is usually transmitted from infected animals to susceptible animals through direct or close indirect contact. Airborne transmission and through infected pastures or fomites are possible but uncommon. There is no evidence of vertical transmission of RPV.

Species susceptibility

- Highly susceptible: Domestic cattle, water buffalo, yak, wildebeest kudu, eland, giraffe, warthogs
- Low susceptible (with milder clinical sign or subclinical infection): Pigs, goats, sheep
- Dead end host: Camelidae family (no role in RPV transmission)

Clinical signs observed in affected animals

The incubation period ranges from 3 to 15 days depending on the virus strain and exposure level. Clinical signs of rinderpest have not been seen since 2001. A milder form of the disease, with the potential to regain classical characteristics, used to occur in association with endemic situations in East Africa.[2]

Classical acute or epizootic form

- Clinical disease is characterized by an acute febrile attack within which prodromal and erosive phases can be distinguished.
- Prodromal period (time between onset of fever and first appearance of oral lesions) lasts on average 3 days.
  - Affected animals develop a pyrexia of between 40°C and 41.5°C (104°F and 106.7°F) together with partial anorexia, depression, reduction of rumination, constipation, lowered milk production, increase of respiratory and cardiac rate, congestion of visible mucosa, slight serous to mucopurulent ocular and nasal discharges, and drying of the muzzle.
- Erosive phase with development of necrotic mouth lesions:

- o At height of fever: flecks of necrotic epithelium appear on the lower lip and gum and in rapid succession may appear on the upper gum and dental pad, on the underside of the tongue, on the cheeks and cheek papillae and on the hard palate; erosions or blunting of the cheek papillae.
  - o Necrotic foci can fuse to form larger patches; material works loose giving rise to shallow, nonhemorrhagic mucosal erosions.
- Gastrointestinal signs appear when the fever drops or about 1 to 2 days after the onset of mouth lesions—diarrhea is usually copious and watery at first; later may contain mucus, blood, and shreds of epithelium accompanied, in severe cases, by tenesmus.
- Diarrhea or dysentery leads to dehydration, abdominal pain, abdominal respiration, and weakness.
- In terminal stages of the illness, animals may become recumbent for 24 to 48 hours prior to death; death usually occurs 6 to 12 days following onset of fever.
- Deaths will occur but mortality rate will be variable and may be expected to rise as the virus gains progressive access to large numbers of susceptible animals—depending on the strain of RPV, initial mortality rates may be as low as 10% to 20% or in the order of 90% in highly susceptible animals. Animals in areas with endemic PPR may show lower mortality and resistance to RPV.
- Some animals die while showing severe necrotic lesions, high fever, and diarrhea, and others die after a sharp fall in body temperature, often to subnormal values.
- In rare cases, clinical signs regress by day 10 and recovery occurs by days 20 to 25.

Peracute Form

- No prodromal signs except high fever (> 40–42°C/104–107.6°F), sometimes congested mucous membranes, and death within 2 to 3 days.
- This form occurs in highly susceptible young and newborn animals.

Mild Subacute or Endemic Form

- Clinical signs limited to one or more of the classic signs.
- Usually no associated diarrhea.
- May show a slight, serous, ocular, or nasal secretion.
- Fever: variable, short-lived (3–4 days) and not very high (38–40°C/100.4–104°F).
- No actual depression; animals may continue to graze, water, and trek.
- Low-or-no mortality, except in highly susceptible species (buffalo, giraffe, eland, and lesser kudu)
  - o In these wild species: fever, nasal discharge, typical erosive stomatitis, gastroenteritis, and death.

Atypical form

- Irregular pyrexia and mild-or-no diarrhea
  - o Fever may remit slightly in the middle of the erosive period, and
  - o 2 to 3 days later, return rapidly to normal accompanied by a quick resolution of the mouth lesions, a halt to the diarrhea and an uncomplicated convalescence
- The lymphotropic nature of RPV leads to immunosuppression and favors recrudescence of latent infections and/or increased susceptibility to other infectious agents.

LESIONS

- Either areas of necrosis and erosions, or congestion and hemorrhage in the mouth, intestines and upper respiratory tracts.
- Highly engorged or gray discoloration of abomasum (epithelial necrosis of mucous membrane); pyloric region severely affected and shows congestion, petechiation, and edema of the submucosa.
- Rumen, reticulum, and omasum usually unaffected; necrotic plaques are occasionally encountered on the pillars of the rumen.
- Enlarged and edematous lymph nodes.
- White necrotic foci in Peyer's patches; lymphoid necrosis and sloughing leaves the supporting architecture engorged or blackened.
- Linear engorgement and blackening of the crests of the folds of the mecum, colon, and rectum ("Zebra striping").
- Typically the carcass of the dead animal is dehydrated, emaciated, and soiled.
- Histologically, evidence of lymphoid and epithelial necrosis accompanied by viral associated syncytia and intracytoplasmic inclusions.
- In milder form of RP, most domestic animals escape development of erosions:
  - Some may develop slight congestion of mucous membranes and small, focal areas of raised, whitish epithelial necrosis may be found on the lower gum (no larger than a pin head); possibly a few eroded cheek papillae.
- In milder form of RP in wild animals:
  - African buffaloes infected with milder RPV have demonstrated enlarged peripheral lymph nodes, plaque-like keratinized skin lesions and keratoconjunctivitis.
  - Lesser kudus were similarly affected with blindness due to severe keratoconjunctivitis but no diarrhea.
  - Eland also showed necrosis and erosions of the buccal mucosa together with dehydration and emaciation.

Differential Diagnosis

Cattle

- Bovine viral diarrhea/mucosal disease
- Malignant catarrhal fever
- Infectious bovine rhinotracheitis
- Foot and mouth disease
- Papular stomatitis
- Jembrana disease
- Vesicular stomatitis
- Contagious bovine pleuropneumonia
- Theileriosis (East Coast fever)
- Salmonellosis
- Necrobacillosis
- Paratuberculosis
- Arsenic poisoning

Small ruminants

- Peste des petits ruminants
- Nairobi sheep disease
- Contagious caprine pleuropneumonia
- Pasteurellosis

Swine

- Campylobacter spp.
- Brachyspira hyodyesntereiae
- Salmonellosis

CASE CONFIRMATION

RP should be suspected when a susceptible animal shows clinical signs consistent with "stomatitis-enteritis syndrome" and where these signs cannot be ascribed to another disease compatible with "stomatitis-enteritis syndrome" by clinical or epidemiologic investigation, thereby corresponding to the WOAH Code definition of "potential case."[3] The occurrence of a potential case should draw special attention if it is linked to identified risks such as proximity to facilities holding RPV-containing material.

A "potential case" can evolve into a "suspected case" when.

1. A potential case for which other diseases compatible with "stomatitis-enteritis syndrome" has been ruled out by clinical and laboratory investigation; or
2. A potential case which has given a positive reaction in a diagnostic test for RPV conducted outside of a WOAH Reference Laboratory for RP; or
3. The detection of RPV-specific antibodies that are not a consequence of vaccination in a susceptible animal without clinical signs.

For a "suspected case" to be confirmed, a FAO/WOAH Reference Laboratory for RP must either.

1. Isolate and identify RPV from a susceptible animal or a product derived from that animal; or
2. Isolate viral antigen or viral RNA specific to RPV in samples from a susceptible animal; or
3. Identify antibodies to RPV that are not a consequence of vaccination
4. Identify a susceptible animal with either epidemiologic links to a confirmed or suspected outbreak of RP or clinical signs consistent with recent infection with RPV.

EXPECTATIONS FROM NORTH AMERICAN PRACTITIONERS AND VETERINARY EDUCATORS

While RP has been successfully eradicated for over a decade, it remains crucial to monitor both the disease and its virus. These should be included in the differential diagnosis for diseases with similar clinical signs. It is imperative to sustain awareness about the disease among animal health authorities, field veterinarians, and farmers. Veterinarians and livestock farmers must stay updated on the current eradication status, including the number of investigated suspected cases.

Additionally, it is essential for veterinary students to understand the disease and its historical impact as part of their disease awareness education. To achieve this, there is a national mandate to incorporate RP into the standard veterinary curriculum. This curriculum should be regularly reviewed and updated to ensure that future veterinarians are well informed about this disease.

This study provides a comprehensive overview of RP with the list of clinical signs of the disease, etiology, and preventive measures.

CLINICS CARE POINTS

- Understanding Rinderpest, Prevention, Emergency Preparedness, International collaboration, Public Awareness Campaigns.

ACKNOWLEDGEMENT

The authors acknowledge the valuable efforts of FAO and WOAH along with other international organizations and national veterinary services, to eradicate rinderpest from the face of the earth. The authors would also like to thank Dr Samia Metwally, Dr Juan Lubroth, and Dr Keith Sumption (FAO); and, from WOAH Dr Kazuaki Miyagishima, Dr Gideon Bruckner, Dr Keith Hamilton, Ms Tianna Brand and Dr Kazutoshi Matsuo, who all helped advance the post-eradication roadmap during their time at the organization. Finally, the authors express their gratitude to the FAO-WOAH Joint Advisory Committee on rinderpest for their valuable contributions during the post-rinderpest era.

DISCLOSURE

The authors have nothing to disclose.

REFERENCES

1. Roeder P, Mariner J, Kock R. 'Rinderpest: the veterinary perspective on eradication'. Philosophical transactions of the Royal Society of London. Series B, Biological Sciences 2013;368(1623):20120139.
2. World Organisation for Animal Health. Rinderpest, Technical disease card. 2020. Available at: www.woah.org/app/uploads/2021/03/rinderpest.pdf. [Accessed 30 October 2023].
3. World Organisation for Animal Health. Infection with rinderpest virus, terrestrial animal health Code. Paris: WOAH; 2022. Available at: https://www.woah.org/en/what-we-do/standards/codes-and-manuals/terrestrial-code-online-access/?id=169&L=1&htmfile=chapitre_rinderpest.htm.
4. Vallat B. Editorial : The Odyssey of Rinderpest Eradication. OIE Bulletin 2011; 2011(2):1–2.
5. Hamilton K, Visser D, Evans B, et al. Identifying and Reducing Remaining Stocks of Rinderpest Virus. Emerg Infect Dis 2015;21(12):2117.
6. Budke CM, Pfeiffer DU, Jones BA, et al. Sequestration and Destruction of Rinderpest Virus-Containing Material 10 Years after Eradication. Emerg Infect Dis 2022; 28(9):1895–8.
7. Myers L, Metwally S, Marrana M, et al. Global Rinderpest Action Plan – Rinderpest is eradicated but not forgotten. Rome, FAO and OIE. 2018. Available at: https://www.fao.org/documents/card/en/c/ca1965en.